T0374477

Killer Diseases of Women

A Woman's Guide to Life-Threatening Diseases

Prem K. Bhandari

iUniverse, Inc.
New York Bloomington

Killer Diseases of Women
A Woman's Guide to Life-Threatening Diseases

iUniverse books may be ordered through booksellers or by contacting:

iUniverse
1663 Liberty Drive
Bloomington, IN 47403
www.iuniverse.com
1-800-Authors (1-800-288-4677)

ISBN: 978-1-4502-2655-4 (pbk)
ISBN: 978-1-4502-2657-8 (cloth)
ISBN: 978-1-4502-2656-1 (ebk)

Library of Congress Control Number: 2010909479

Printed in the United States of America

iUniverse rev. date: 8/2/2010

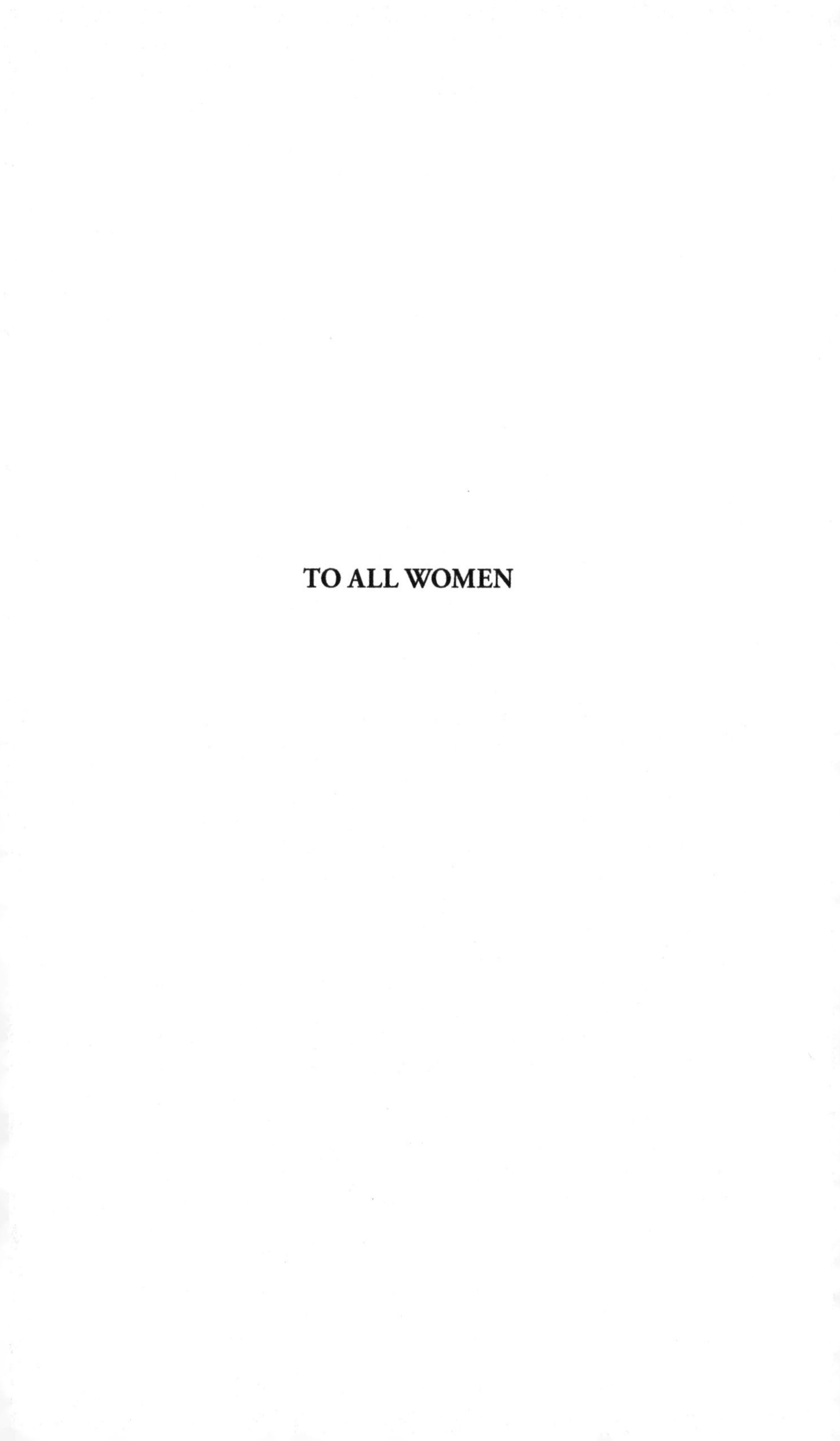

TO ALL WOMEN

Contents

INTRODUCTION

Focusing on diseases that are fatal to women is a recent phenomenon, and the researchers are becoming more aware of the specialized healthcare needs of women. Women don't have to become dependent upon the availability of healthcare when needed, even though they pay their healthcare premiums regularly and are eligible to claim it; instead they should try to avoid seeking healthcare through taking precautionary measures and self health management. 2004 figures reveal that 1,215,947 women died in the USA of all diseases combined in comparison to 1,181,668 men during the same period. This tells you why women should arm themselves with some understanding of their bodies and the diseases that afflict them.

Medical knowledge is an evolving science which has not been able to pinpoint the exact causes of most deadly diseases, so far. The cures have been reactive measures in response to diagnosis of diseases, and increasingly more suitable cures are being found and instituted. Even if the exact causes and the respective cures to bring satisfactory outcomes are discovered, women should not depend solely on the third party to cure some deadly disease which has inflicted them. Women should prepare themselves for all eventualities, even for misdiagnosis which cost at least 200,000 deaths each year in the USA alone.

For more than fifty years in different regions of the world, including where sign-language was the only means to communicate, I have witnessed that knowledge of diseases, wellness measures, disease prevention, medical help, and other protective attention were at the minimum level for women. Until recently, in most of the world, women were considered only as a possession. Even in the well to do households, women's health was never an over riding priority over some daily routine. I have watched men leaving the house for some errand or social reason leaving the unattended wife in pain and near death. There are millions of cases like this throughout the world, and enforcement of social ethical values does not travel far.

For cultural, economic, and social reasons very few women have any 'voice', which renders them weak in being heard and in receiving appropriate attention for their healthcare needs. What really works is 'education'. If all women know the symptoms and the root causes of the life threatening diseases, they will be well prepared to take care of themselves in the first place, and secondly they will be able to deal with the medical community in the most effective manner. They will have confidence to deal with any disease and any situation related to it.

All women should arm themselves with some knowledge of their physical anatomy, functions of each organ, and other health related pertinent information which will help them to familiarize themselves with various symptoms of many life threatening health conditions. Knowledge of symptoms can save women's life from most diseases; it will make them concerned and compel them to take preventive measures right away. Most women die of various diseases primarily because of lack of knowledge; they fail to recognize the symptoms, and fail to effectively communicate with the medical community. If the condition progresses, they don't know how to express it specifically and what to do in the given circumstances. On the other hand, few doctors really know what the patient is suffering from, how to recognize the symptoms, how to diagnose, and what should be the treatment. Most of them work on an educated guess based on their individual education, experience, capabilities, intelligence, and interest in the patient. Most of them are good at writing a prescription, calling for tests, recommending surgeries, etc.

Women should always remember that in America the healthcare system is based on business model under somewhat competitive marketplace settings which compels the medical community as a whole to generate and increase revenues annually. Therefore, no matter how good the intentions happen to be, the medical community generates as many dollars as possible to survive, to pay high salaries, to produce higher revenues for the directors and shareholders, etc. Patients become customers of the medical community who would not mind cultivating them, intensively and extensively, to maximize their profits, and the healthy population becomes 'potential business prospects' for the future.

Additionally, due to the fear of law-suits, today the doctors are compelled to order a battery of tests on your body before diagnosing the health problem. Today, healthcare is bound by insurance laws, profits, and safeguards against libel, in combination with incompetence, medical errors, unnecessary procedures and costs, and carelessness. We seem to have created a scenario where we seek others to tell what is wrong with us, instead of knowing ourselves. We outsource our decisions which are crucial to our wellbeing and longevity. Of course, when health problems get out of control and become life or death situation, we are obliged to let the medical community decide, which should be in the column of exceptions only.

Health problems just don't appear suddenly, it takes a long time for a serious health problem to emerge and much before that several symptoms start waving the red flag. Most doctors may not consider your symptoms to be serious and are most likely to provide you with an instant relief with a prescription. Women need to recognize these red flags of warning which should trigger immediate remedial actions on their part. If women learn to know their body and the symptoms of each killer disease, or non-killer disease, they may never have to depend on the medical help for 90% of the time, because they will start taking precautionary measures right from the beginning when the symptoms first appear.

To manage your life you have to manage your health even during the time you are under medical treatment. Knowledgeable and prepared women patients will ask the right questions, understand the buzzwords, nuances, and get somewhat better medical health. The medical doctors and the staff when dealing with knowledgeable women patients will be much more alert and treat them with a lot more respect, attention, and discipline. They will be refreshing upon the educational material which helped them get the license to practice medicine. Most of them are not aware of the new medical breakthroughs, and knowledgeable patients can drive them to keep up with the new developments. After all, you pay an enormous amount of health insurance premium every month and your visit to the doctor is not a social one or a pastime; you want the best out of your each visit besides getting better faster.

The contents of Killer Diseases of Women will acquaint you with the most deadly diseases, symptoms, causes, some preventions and recommendations wherever possible. I have tried to use a very simple language for women from all walks of life to understand it. If you succeed in understanding it, you will end up knowing more than most medical professionals you come across. You will be armed with an advantage of having the knowledge and talking points, and will understand your condition and the medical treatment each step of the way. Most likely, you will reduce your dependency on the medical community by as much as 90%.

Why do women need to learn about various killer diseases when we have world class healthcare system? Why can't the medical community look after women when women need them? Yes, they will definitely look after all patients. All women should look at the other side of the coin. In spite of the world class healthcare system in the United States, about 35 million women suffer from serious digestive problems and about 120,000 die, about 12 million get hospitalized, and about 1,000,000 get disabled yearly in the United States. These digestive diseases are intestinal hernias (mostly inguinal), liver diseases including cirrhosis, constipation, diverticulosis, gallbladder diseases, gastritis, esophageal disorders, hemorrhoids, infectious diarrhea, irritable bowel syndrome, etc.

Apart from the disastrous effects of digestive diseases, we can add several million more incidents, hospitalization, deaths, and disability related to heart disease, stroke, various cancers, septicemia, COPD, diabetes, dementia, influenza, misdiagnoses, etc. All women should acquaint themselves with the symptoms, causes, and preventive measures to live a healthier and longer life.

Reading *Killer Diseases of Women* will make you aware of the importance of self healthcare management, and the best way to do it, with having periodic check ups through the help of knowledgeable medical community. But your knowledge of your own body, health condition, symptoms of disease, and willingness to manage any health problem, including the medically assisted ones, will save you from disability or death, and prolong your life. Knowing your body, recognizing symptoms of various diseases, communicating with the medical community effectively, and taking the recommended precautions will reduce your medical visits by at least 80% if not more, save an enormous amount of time and money, and improve your health and quality of life in general.

Through *Killer Diseases of Women*, you will learn to recognize symptoms and the emergence of many diseases, to deliberate possible solutions, to suitably modify your lifestyle for avoiding them or healing from them, and to be able to appropriately deal with the medical community in the most effective and meaningful manner that benefits you.

Prem K. Bhandari has authored "Heal & Prevent Stroke & Heart Disease", "Psychological Traits Link to Eczema", and numerous policy papers on the self management of nation's major health threats. Over the span of 50 years, through observations, in depth conversations, surveys, and research in Asia, Europe, and North America, he has concluded that 80 to 90 percent of life-threatening diseases are preventable through knowledge and recognition of symptoms and taking timely remedial measures.

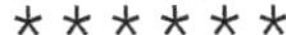

CANCER

Cancer is described as a blight that spreads destructively within the body. Cancer starts when a cell is somehow altered resulting in its abnormal behavior and out of control growth. Under normal conditions, human body continuously gives birth to new cells to replace the old, damaged, and dead cells. This process of the death and birth of cells is a continuous one in our body. In scientific language, when the cells divide and new cells are born, it is called ***mitosis.*** On the other hand, the process of destroying and discarding the old and damaged cells is known as ***apoptosis.***

Cancer is not a single disease, but a combination of several diseases affecting most parts of the body. Almost all types of cancers are life threatening and should be taken very seriously. The most fundamental cause of cancer is the damage or alteration of the genetic code in a healthy cell nucleus. This damage or alteration is caused by certain elements called ***carcinogens*** (cancer causing). Cell alteration or damage can result because of external or internal factors. The ***external factors*** are pollution and cancer causing elements which can damage the DNA in the nucleus of the cell, causing birth and mutation of abnormal cells which form a colony, penetrate various layers and enter the bloodstream, and then spread to other parts of the body. The ***internal factors*** are just errors occurring, like in any other gigantic and complicated system, in the body which contains about 3 trillion cells of which about 10 million die every second. A huge number! Often, a cell gets damaged, or happens to be abnormal or week and mutates, which damages other healthy cells. Under healthy and normal conditions, body's immune system will identify such abnormal and mutating cells and destroy them before they multiply.

Most cancer occur as a result of the external factors which are environmental and lifestyle related. Cancers of lung, breast, pancreas, kidneys, stomach, uterus, bladder, and skin are linked to the type of food we eat, and the chemicals, toxins, infections, and poisons in the environment we live, breathe, work, and grow our foods in. Many substances in our environment and food intake have been identified as carcinogens. Carcinogens include a variety of chemicals, gases, dangerous substances found in the water, air, and foods, tobacco smoke, industrial fumes, auto fumes, herbicides, pesticides, paints, nuclear radiation, excessive exposure to sunshine, radio active waste, x rays, various viruses, detergents, metals in the air, etc.

Some time ago, The American Cancer Society declared seven warning signs of cancer:

*Change in bowel or bladder habits.
*A sore that wouldn't heal.
*Unusual bleeding or discharge.
*Thickening or lump in the breast or elsewhere.
*Indigestion or difficulty in swallowing.
*Obvious change in a wart or mole.
*Nagging cough or hoarseness.

These are certainly the most obvious symptoms of the presence of tumor and/or cancer in an area of the body; however, in the following pages you will find unique ones attributable to specific organs.

DNA controls the process of mitosis and apoptosis. If for some reason, the DNA is damaged, the genes that control may not function properly. Cells that act like stoplights during cell growth and division may breakdown, which may lead to the development and growth of ***oncogenes (tumor causing)*** which stimulate uncontrolled cell growth. Damage to DNA may lead to the destruction of the protective genes, called ***suppressor genes,*** which prevent abnormal cells from growing in to tumors.

Radiation, chemicals, toxins, sunlight, tobacco smoke, virus infections, and the genetic makeup can damage the DNA, where our genetic material and program is stored. When DNA is damaged and an uncontrolled cell growth occurs, cancer cells invade the body. Tumor is formed when cancer cells form a cluster or abnormal tissues. Tumors are like cancer fortresses and affect various organs like breasts, lungs, intestinal tract, bladder, etc. From an established tumor, cancer cells can spread to the surrounding tissue and to the distant parts of the body via the blood stream, a condition known as ***metastasis***. If the cells travel from an established tumor, say, in the bladder and metastasize to the liver, similar tumors may appear in the liver. The tumors in the liver will have bladder cancer cells, despite the fact that they are in the liver. Each type of cancer has a unique characteristic, even within a particular cancer type, and its behavior is unique in itself.

The most prominent challenges for the scientists are why cells divide, what causes cell aging and death, and why cancer cells damage a particular component of gene in the nucleus of cells under attack. Normally, a cell divides about 50 times before it stops reproducing and its death, and this upper limit is famously known as ***Hay Flick limit*** (Leonard Hay Flick discovered this during his research). All cells age, stop reproducing, and die. Different body cells have different life span. For example: ***granulocytes***, a type of white blood cell, lives between 13 to 20 days, ***red blood cells*** live about 120 days, ***keratinocyte*** (one of skin cell types) has a lifespan of 14 to 28 days, etc. However, there are certain types of cells which will not die as long as you are alive, and they are the cells of the heart muscle, and neurons in the brain.

Aging process of the cells in our body has drawn attention and interest of all scientists around the world but, though several theories are out there, no exact scientific explanation has been found. Although not absolutely scientific, yet somewhat convincing hypothesis have been made in this regard.

1) One is that the cells get damaged by continuous exposure to and accumulation of environmental toxins, like fumes, exhausts, chemicals, poisons, etc, and over time certain cells start dying from it.

2) Genetic influence in destroying the cells after a predetermined period of time, which happens at the time of cell division. It's a hypothesis which claims that at certain cell divisions, the end of the chromosome, called ***telomere***, is torn, which may be the signal for the cell to cease dividing.

3) The ***free radicals*** in our body could be the reason why our cells get damaged and/or die. Free radicals are molecules with one electron missing in them, and if they enter a cell, the electrons from molecules of the healthy cells are pulled out and get attached to them (free radicals), which destabilize and damage the healthy cells. Surprisingly cancer cells can divide and reproduce without aging.

RECOMMENDATIONS

*Stop tobacco smoking, tobacco chewing, and tobacco environment.
*Drink alcohol only in moderation.
*Avoid excessive exposure to ultra violet rays of the sun, and use the sunscreen while out in the sun.
*Get cancer screening, but not often (accumulative effects of x-rays cause cancer).

*Keep your body active and in good shape by exercising regularly.
*Adopt a healthy diet and lifestyle.
*Avoid exposure to ***carcinogens*** by staying away from the industrial zones, auto-fumes, cleaning detergents, spraying products, chemicals, herbicides, pesticides, weed killers, nuclear stations, high tension electric transmission cables, etc.
*Follow safety guidelines whenever near the cancer causing agents (carcinogens).

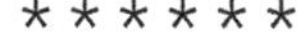

CANCER IN UPPER BODY

BREAST CANCER

About 218.000 new cases of breast cancer appear on the scene each year, and about 42, 000 women die of it. It is one third of all cancers in women. The incidence of death by breast cancer in women is just behind colorectal and lung cancers. More than half a million women die of breast cancer, worldwide, after being diagnosed, each year when an unknown number die in the absence of healthcare, regular check ups, and records. Breast cancer is more treatable than colorectal and lung cancers.

Women's breasts go through temporary changes each month during menstruation, and a lump may form. About 90% of these lumps are non cancerous. Lumps may form in the lobules or in the ducts. ***Lobules*** are small sacs where the milk is produced, and the ***ducts*** are from where the milk is carried to the nipples.

The starting point of breast cancer is when a tumor is formed. Some tumors are strictly local and do not spread to other areas; they are called ***benign***. The other kind of tumor invades nearby tissues, and is cancerous, called ***malignant***. There are several types of breast cancer; however, ***lobular carcinoma*** and ***ductal carcinoma*** are the most prominent ones. All cancers can spread to other parts of the body, called metastasizing of cancer. Different types of breast cancers grow and spread at a different rate and speed. Some are slower than others. Cancer spreads through the blood stream and lymphatic system. The ***lymphatic system*** is the conveyor of the lymph (yellowish liquid containing the white blood cells) from the cells to the blood stream and by which the white blood cells are produced to respond to the inflammation and foreign bacteria. The lymphatic system is comprised of lymph glands, vessels, and sinuses through which lymph is carried to the blood stream.

METASTATIC BREAST CANCER

When cancer spreads from the breast area to other parts of the body, like brain, leg, heart, etc is called metastatic breast cancer.

INFLAMMATORY BREAST CANCER

When the cancer develops in patches rather than in lumps, and invades nearby skin, it changes the color of the breast, and causes itching. The breast feels harder and firmer than before, warm to touch, and sometime ulcerated.

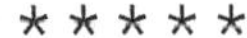

SPREADING OF BREAST CANCER

Breast cancer spreads by way of the lymphatic system and the blood stream. Once the cancer cells reach the blood stream, they can travel to other parts of the body, including the brain, and metastasize.

Each breast is surrounded by 12 to 25 glandular lobes which

contain ***alveolus*** (small sacs) that produce milk. Each lobe has ducts, called lactiferous ducts, to carry milk to the nipple. Each breast is also equipped with different lymph node chains which control the drainage of non-blood liquids from designated locations in the breast and around it. For example, the ***brachial nodes*** drain lymph liquids from most of the arm, the ***pectoral nodes*** drain from most of the breast and anterior chest, the ***sub-scapular nodes*** drain **part** of the arm and the posterior chest, the ***mid-axillary nodes*** act as the central draining nodes for the pectoral, brachial, and the sub-scapular nodes; and the ***internal mammary nodes*** drain the mammary lobes.

Lumps on the breasts can be cancerous or non cancerous, and their causes to appear may be varied. Similarly, fluid filled cyst on the breast may appear and the reasons may be different in each occurrence. In each and every case, including flat skin or some dark spot appearing on the breast, doctor should be contacted without delay for a thorough check up. The prudence is in identifying even the remotest indicators, if there are any, at an early stage.

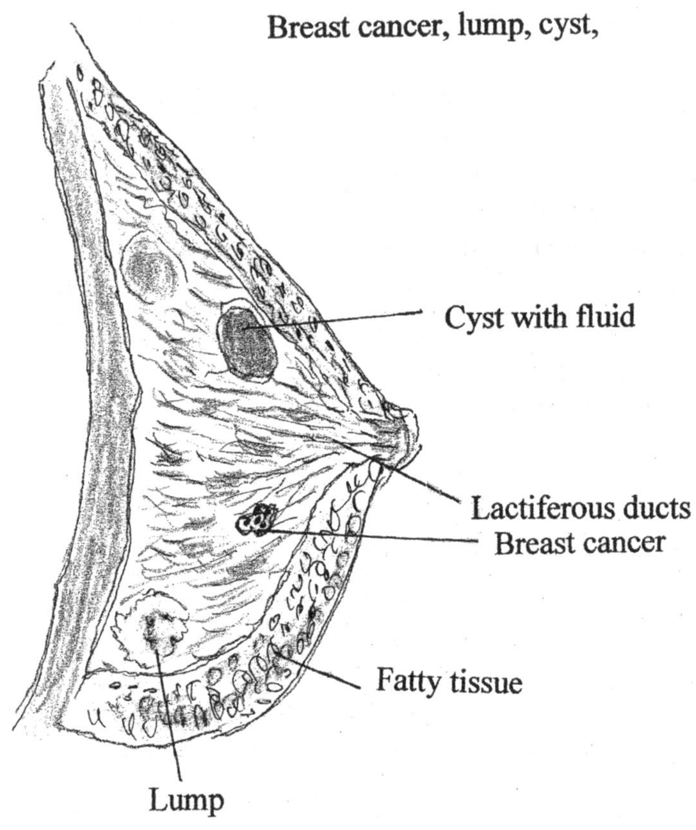

The Lymphatic system is the most common route for cancer cells to cause breast cancer. Any obstruction within the lymph nodes and the ducts can cause blockages which in turn can produce some inflammation and an invitation to cell damage, and cancer.

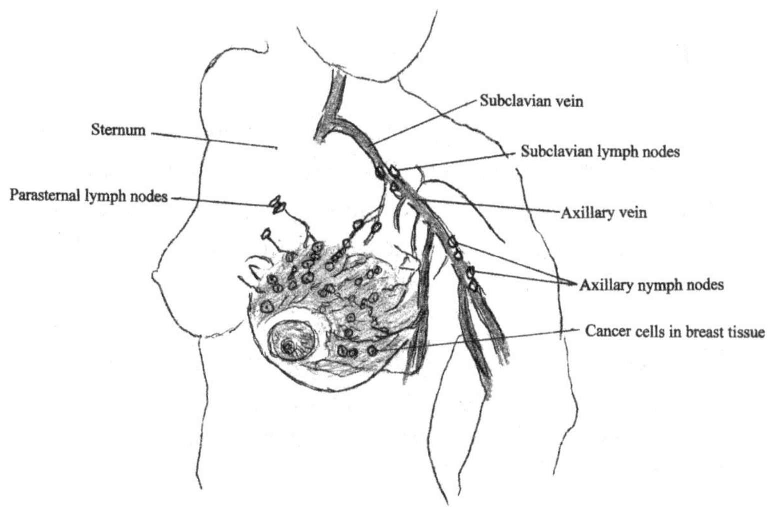

BREAST CANCER RECURRENCES

Sometime, cancer reappears after showing signs of complete healing. The recurrence may be local or distant. 1) Local recurrence will indicate small lumps and skin rash under the skin. 2) Distant recurrence will be identified by swollen lymph in the armpit, and/or on the side of the neck, and/or above the collar bones.

SYMPTOMS

*Swelling or lump in the breast.
*Swelling in the armpits (lymph nodes).
*Clear or bloody nipple discharge.
*Pain in the nipples.
*Inverted nipples.
*Scaly or pitted skin on the nipples.
*Pain in the breast.
*Change in the contour, color, expansion or flattening of breast.
*Persistent tenderness of the breast.

CAUSES

*The most significant facts are advancing age, and the family history of female patients. Women whose mother, sister, or daughter, have had cancer are more likely to get breast cancer. Genes do play an important role and researchers think that they are linked to the familial breast cancer.

*Women who have passed the age 50, and are in menopausal stage are more likely to get breast cancer than the ones who are not in that category. African women are more likely to get breast cancer than the Caucasian.

*Researchers believe there is a strong link between breast cancer and hormones. Women with higher exposure to ***estrogen*** (female hormone) are more likely to get breast cancer. Estrogen signals the cells to divide. Excessive cell divisions produce abnormal cells which become cancerous.

*Risk of breast cancer is increased if a woman started menstruating before the age 13, or stops menstruating after the age 55 or her menstrual cycle is longer or shorter than normal.

*Women who take hormone replacement therapy, or take birth control pills, or have been exposed to heavy doses of radiation therapy may be at a higher risk of getting breast cancer.

*High fat diets, obesity, tobacco smoking, alcohol abuse, stress, pollutants, pesticides, herbicides, or genetic defect are the most prominent risk factors for the breast cancer.

*Each cell in our body has a nucleus where the genetic code

resides. We are all controlled by the program written on these genetic codes. Under normal conditions, the old cells die and are replaced by the new ones in our body, which is an ongoing natural process, but as time goes on this process can create mutations. Mutations are a departure from the norm with a slight change in genes within the cell. Over time, such mutations take place in the cells of our body. This causes certain genes to get turned off, and others to turn on. This changes the cell itself. The changed cells gain ability to keep dividing over time without control and producing more unique cells like them, forming a tumor.

RECOMMENDATIONS

*Check your breasts each day during shower or bath. Women above 50 should have a complete exam periodically without over exposure to x-rays and other scans. Regular self and medical examinations are important for early detection, because if cancer reaches on the skin of the breast, it may have progressed to an advanced stage.
*If you have a family history of breast cancer or other cancers then talk to your doctor about the best way to manage menopause without estrogen pills.
*Ask your doctor if you should take birth control pills before taking them.
*Your diet should mainly consist of grains, fruits, vegetables, legumes, lentils, and lots of water.

*Eliminate fats and fried foods from your diet.
*Ask your doctor for the right dosages of vitamin supplements.
*No dairy products, except a small amount of certain low fat yogurt and cheese should be in your diet, if you have been diagnosed with cancer.

*Minimize exposure to MRI, x-ray, mammogram, scans, etc to an absolute necessity.

*Your doctor should determine if the hormone receptors are present. Receptors are the interpreters of the messages received from the hormones. Receptors can influence turning on and turning off cell growth in the breast.
*No animal flesh should be in your diet.
*No manufactured sugar should be in your diet. All sugar requirements should be met through fruits, vegetables, nuts, seeds, grains, etc.

*Maintain healthy weight levels.
*Complete bowel movements on daily basis must become a routine
*Adopt a happy attitude, peaceful and social lifestyle without anxieties
*Let the body sweat regularly, allowing it to drain out toxins, waste, and foreign elements

*Mothers should breast feed their babies for as long as there is milk in the breasts. Milk should not remain in the breasts because the body is geared to producing milk during that time, and the stagnant milk in the lactiferous ducts can put mothers at a high risk of breast cancer in the future.
*Take plenty of rest each and every day, and maintain regular sleeping schedule.

Certain foods can make your body healthier, improve metabolism, improve the immune system, and help you reduce the risk of breast cancer. Therefore, choice of lifestyle and diet play an important role in preventing the breast cancer to occur, or return.

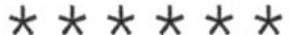

HEARTBURN AND ESOPHAGEAL CANCER

Heartburn is linked to esophageal cancer, and it has nothing to do with the heart; it's just a name for burning sensation in the esophagus. After chewing, the food travels through the esophagus to the stomach which empties it in to the intestinal tract. It takes anywhere from 2 to 5 hours for the food to travel from mouth to the intestinal tract. If food is not chewed properly, or the food is swallowed too quickly, or too much food is pushed down the throat in to the esophagus, it can cause heartburn. The food intake requires chewing properly, should be swallowed slowly, and only small quantities of food should be eaten at a single time to allow enough enzymes from the mouth glands to accompany the well chewed food to the esophagus. If the quantity of food is more than the sufficient amount of enzymes generated in the mouth or if too much food is swallowed in a very short time then the food will sit at the bottom of the esophagus and enter very slowly in to the stomach through a muscular valve called ***esophageal sphincter.***

Esophageal sphincter opens up to allow the food to enter slowly and in increments. If the sphincter remains open for a long time due to congestion, the stomach juices can reflux and seep in to the esophagus giving a burning sensation which is commonly known as ***"heartburn"***. Esophageal sphincter, the muscular valve, can also become weak if it is stretched too much or remains open too long, which results from large chunks of insufficiently chewed food, as well as too much food passing through it on regular basis. Stretched and weak esophageal sphincter will not close properly and the stomach juices will seep in regularly causing heartburn sensation.

The sensation of heartburn is also linked to the excessive amounts of caffeine and ***Theo bromine***, (a kind of poison found in coffee, tea, cocoa and some cola), refined carbohydrates (sugars, white bread, pasta), sour drinks, acidic foods, tomatoes, vinegar, and smoking. These foods and some other cause ***gastro-esophageal reflux.*** Heartburn, caused by refluxes, is linked to ***Esophageal Cancer.*** The gastro-esophageal reflux contains a very powerful corrosive acid called ***Hydrochloric Acid*** which can destroy the mucus which protects the lining of esophagus and stomach, giving way to the foreign bodies to colonize inside the lining.

Portions of food, drink, and stomach juices can return to the esophagus from the stomach as a result of

1) Weakened and stretched sphincter valve which connects the esophagus and the stomach.
2) Through over eating.
3) Hiatus hernia.
4) Pregnancy ulcers.
5) Too much or too little stomach acid due to the damage in the stomach lining
6) Lack of folic acid.
7) lack of vitamin A.
8) Food allergies which stimulate histamine release and trigger the secretion of stomach acids.
9) Gas and indigestion caused by insufficient stomach acids, and causing contents to reflux in to the esophagus and irritate its cells, and eventually damage the mucus.
10) Intolerance to milk, beef, citrus, corn, eggs, soy products, etc.
11) There may be other existing problems like: gallbladder stones, stomach ulcers, heart disease, irritable bowel syndrome, etc.

* * * * *

ESOPHAGEAL CANCER

Esophagus is the long tube that runs from throat to the stomach. Tumor can form on the inside wall of the esophagus. The symptoms don't appear until much later when the tumor is well established, which narrows the passage through which food and liquids pass from throat to the stomach. The most prominent symptoms are: difficulty in swallowing solid food initially, and later difficulty with liquids, chronic dry cough, etc. Once the tumor penetrates the lining of the esophagus, it can travel and spread to other parts of the body. Immediate medical help should be sought.

Heartburn is linked to esophageal cancer, and about 10 million women suffer from it, more than 450,000 get hospitalized, and more than 20,000 are disabled every year.

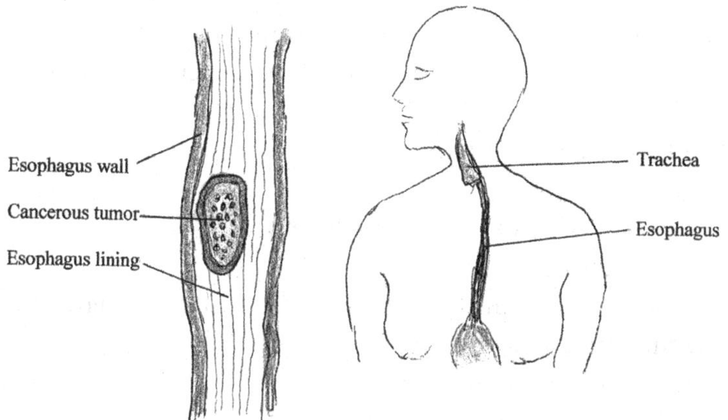

CAUSES

*Over eating and drinking
*Eating too fast and not chewing food properly.
*Eating acidic foods in excess.
*Eating at irregular hours and not maintaining any regular eating schedule.
*Tobacco smoking and exposure to tobacco environment.
*Consuming alcohol excessively.
*Going to bed immediately after eating.
*Stretched sphincter valve which connects the esophagus and the stomach.

*Insufficient quantities of digestive juices which include Hydrochloric Acid.

(Note: ***hydrochloric acid*** is an extremely powerful acid which has a wide range of industrial applications including cleaning of metals, is produced naturally in the stomach. It can burn the stomach lining instantly in the absence of mucus, a slime secreted by the mucous membrane. Hydrochloric acid protects us from harmful bacteria, and is crucial to our digestive process. Food won't get digested properly if sufficient quantity of hydrochloric acid is not there resulting in malnutrition. Also, impaired hydrochloric acid secretion will not be able to provide protection to the body against harmful bacteria. Lower levels of hydrochloric acid allows harmful bacteria to colonize and outnumber the beneficial bacteria)

RECOMMENDATIONS

*Stop smoking tobacco immediately.
*Eat small amounts of food at a time.
*Consume maximum one alcoholic drink per day, if not eliminating it altogether.
*Eat small meals in the evenings.
*Maintain mealtime regularity.
*Chew food thoroughly and swallow it slowly in small portions.
*Last meal of the day should be at least 3 hours before going to bed.
*Drink hot tea or coffee, or warm water after each meal, especially after day's last meal.

*Use two pillows to raise your head while sleeping, so that any reflux during the night remains below the esophagus.
*Make sure that there is no sensation of heartburn or reflux at any time of the day or night.

*Get up from the bed immediately upon any sensation of heartburn or reflux, and wait until it subsides.
*Try your best not to let reflux or heartburn occur in the first place.

LUNG CANCER

Lung cancer is a leading cause of cancer deaths in the United States, and about 73,000 women die of it each year, and over 700,000 die worldwide. About 90% of lung cancer is caused by tobacco smoking and excessive exposure to second hand smoke, while the other causes include exposure to asbestos, radon, and family history. Tobacco smoke contains about 4,000 chemical compounds, and about 400 carbon compounds which include benzene, hydrogen cyanide, nicotine, tar, carbon monoxide, etc. All of these chemicals are cancer causing elements and exposure to them is an invitation to cancer in the lungs and other parts of the body. Tobacco smoking and being in the environment of tobacco smoke (second hand smoke) is an established cancer causing fact. Women who have been treated for lung cancer have about 14% chance to survive after 5 years.

Our two lungs are cone shaped and lie on either side of our chest cavity. They rest on the muscle known as diaphragm and their top part is in the core of the neck. Each lung is surrounded by a thin membrane called pleura. Lungs help us breathe about 12,000 quarts of air each day, of which oxygen is about little less than one-fifth of its volume, and the rest is nitrogen and a trace of other gases. Humans cannot live without oxygen more than a few minutes even though more than half of our body weight is oxygen (water is eight-ninth of oxygen). Therefore, lungs are absolutely essential for humans to be able to breathe and live.

Most commonly, lung cancer begins in the cells that line your lungs. Tobacco smoking causes majority of lung cancers. (Lung cancer also occurs in non-smokers) Tobacco smoke damages the cells that line the lungs. Changes in the lung tissue begin immediately, cell replacement becomes rapid and in the process cells become altered in size, shape, and organization. These altered cells become abnormal and cease to protect, so the underlying tissues become exposed to irritants and carcinogens. Eventually, these abnormal cells grow out of control and start invading deeper tissues.

Regular tobacco smoking damages the cells repeatedly, causing the cells to act abnormally, and eventually cancer may develop. Lungs are full of blood vessels and lymph vessels which provide easy access to the cancer cells to travel to other parts of the body. In many cases, lung cancer may spread to other parts of the body before it can even be detected in the lungs. There are two main types of lung cancer:

1. **Small Cell Lung Cancer** occurs almost exclusively in heavy smokers. It is the most aggressive form of cancer. It is also called the oat cell cancer because under microscope it looks like oat grain. It originates in the central bronchi. It spreads quickly, even before the symptoms are detectable.

2. **Non Small Cell Carcinoma** is an umbrella for several types of lung cancers which include
   ****Squamous cell carcinoma*** usually starts in the cells, which are scale-like, of the central bronchi which are the largest branches of the bronchial tree. It is the second most common type of lung cancer, and accounts for about 30% of all lung cancers.
   ****Adenocarcinoma*** is the most common type

of lung cancer in women smokers and the non smokers. It accounts for about 50% of all lung cancers. It originates along the outer edges of the lung in the small bronchi. It can spread to the spaces between the lungs and the chest wall. Its location makes early detection difficult. Similar type of cancer can appear in the linings of breast, stomach, colon, cervix, and prostate.

***Large cell carcinomas** are a group of cancers that originate along the outer edges of the lungs. They are not very common.

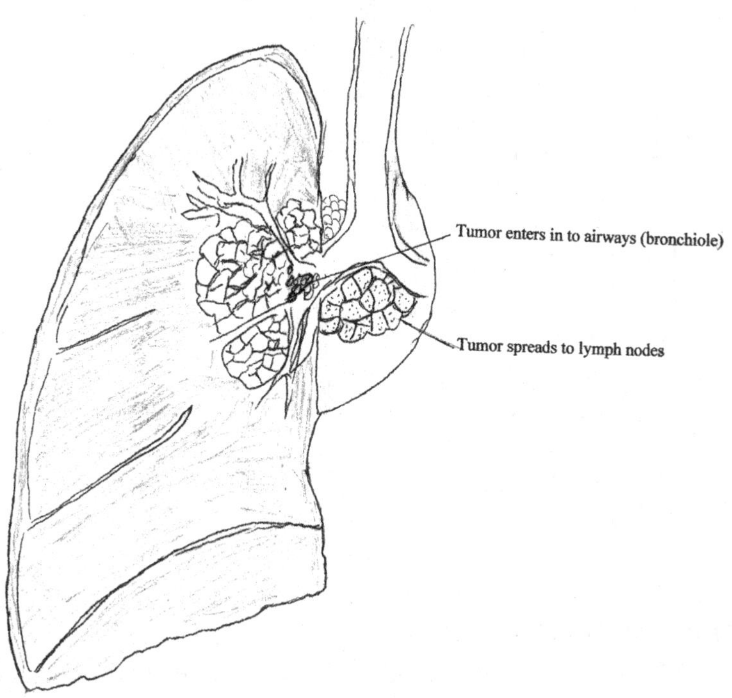

METASTASIS OF LUNG CANCER

Cancer originating from lungs can travel and spread to other parts of the body through the bloodstream. Most likely destinations for lung cancer to establish itself in the other lung, shoulder bone, liver, stomach, and the brain.

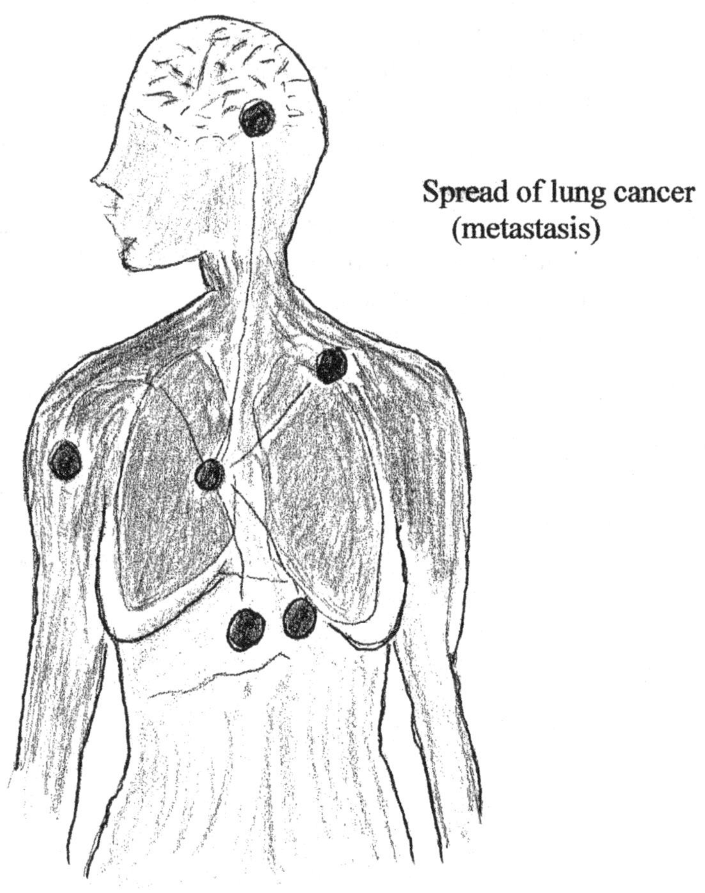

Spread of lung cancer
(metastasis)

RISK FACTORS

*Women who are current smokers, or were smokers at one time have the greatest risk.

*Women are more susceptible to the cancer causing substances in tobacco, because women inhale much more than men do, and women are less likely to quit smoking tobacco.

*Smoking is directly connected to lung cancer. The quantity of tobacco smoke inhaled determines the degree of risk of getting lung cancer.

*Exposure to second hand smoke causes increased risk of lung cancer.

*Exposure to radon gas increases the risk of getting lung cancer. Radon gas is produced naturally by the breakdown of uranium in the soil, water, rocks, and air. Radon gas can get accumulated in your house and increase the risk of lung cancer.

*Family history of lung cancer can be crucial in the determination of your risk factor. Close family members like parents, children, sisters, brothers, and near relatives with lung cancer will increase your risk of getting lung cancer.

*Women with Chronic Obstructive Pulmonary Disease are at high risk of contracting lung cancer.

*Women residing in the industrial, and traffic polluted zones are at increased risk of getting lung cancer.

*Excessive use of alcohol can also increase your risk of getting lung cancer. One drink per day for women is just enough.

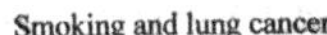

Smoking and lung cancer

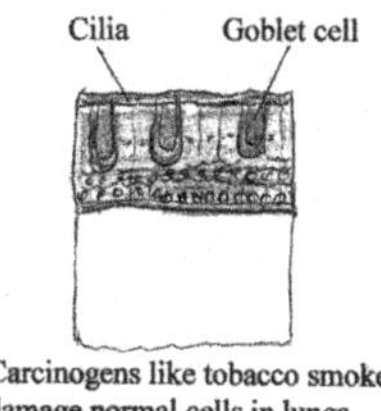

Carcinogens like tobacco smoke damage normal cells in lungs

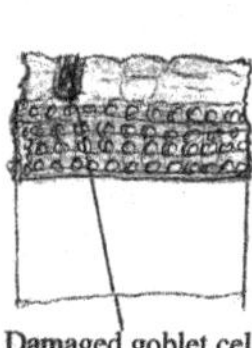

Damaged goblet cell

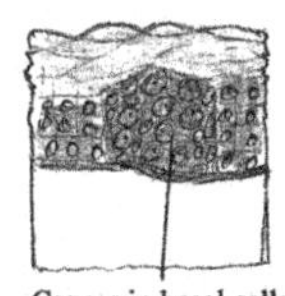

Cancer in basal cells

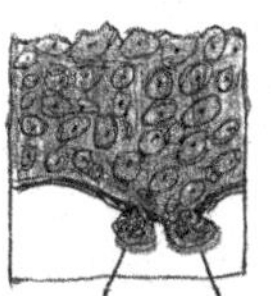

Cancer cells multiply and penetrate the bronchus

RECOMMENDATIONS

*Quit tobacco smoking.
*Avoid tobacco smoke environment.
*Avoid or minimize exposure to heavy automobile traffic areas.
*Avoid exposure to substances like asbestos, silica, herbicides, pesticides, and alike.

*Avoid exposure to fumes containing any kind of metal, or chemical.
*Exercise regularly to allow lungs to breath and fill up with the fresh air.
*Avoid using anti-perspirants because they seem to seal the skin and the sweat glands. Allow your body to sweat so that body dirt, chemicals, and toxins come out through the pores of your skin.
*Eat nutritious food, including several leafy green vegetables and fruits, daily.
*Drink more than 8 glasses of water daily.

*Maintain contact with your doctor.
*Avoid visiting industrial areas.
*Avoid drinking alcohol.
*With the help of your doctor, take vitamin A, C, and E which, according to most researchers, protect the lungs from the harmful effects of carcinogens.
*Maintain regular and sufficient sleeping and resting routines.

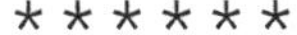

METASTATIC CARCINOMA

Tumors are abnormal growth which may be cancerous. Cancerous tumors have tendency to spread to other parts of the body, which is termed metastasize. Cancer from one location spreads to other locations and ***metastasize*** there and causing a similar type of cancer. There are a few prominent examples of metastasized carcinoma:

LUNG: Metastasizing to the lungs is quite common for many types of cancers which originate elsewhere in the body. The symptoms include: dry cough, cough with bloody sputum, shortness of breath, chest pain, etc.

BONE: Metastasized cancer in the bone originates mostly from breast and lungs. Common symptoms are: pain in the bones, broken bones with minor injury, etc.

BRAIN: Any type of cancer can spread to the brain; however, the most common sources are the lungs and breast cancers. Headache, dizziness, blurred vision, anxiety without any known reason, etc are the common symptoms.

LIVER: Most common cancers to metastasize to the liver are various gastrointestinal cancers, and colon cancer. Common symptoms include weight loss, loss of appetite, jaundice, fever, nausea, swelling of legs (edema), abdominal pain, etc.

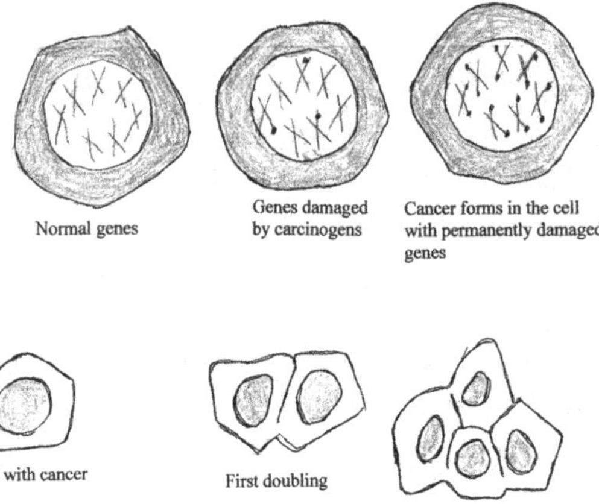

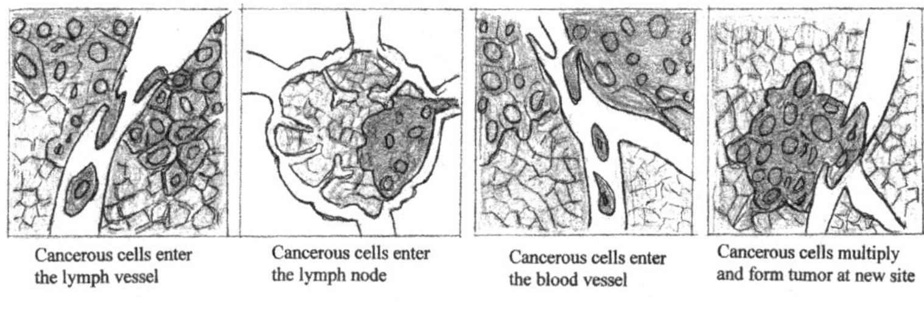

* * * * * *

PANCREATIC DISEASES & CANCER

Pancreas is a small organ, between 4 to 6 inches long, and is located near the stomach. It plays an important role in the digestion of food. It produces a variety of digestive juices which help the body in the digestion of food. There are two kinds of cells in pancreas that are of significance, Endocrine and Exocrine. ***Endocrine cells*** are devoted to hormone regulation, while the ***Exocrine cells*** perform the digestive function. There are 95 Exocrine cells to 1

Endocrine cell. The most prominent digestive juices produced by the pancreas are:

*__*digestive enzymes*__ which go directly in to the gastro-intestinal tract,

*__*bicarbonate*__ which goes directly in to the gastro-intestinal tract, and

*__*insulin*__ which goes directly in to the bloodstream.

When food passes from the stomach to the small intestine through a muscle which acts like a control valve, known as ***pylorus***, pancreas produce and inject additional enzymes:

*__*lipase*__ for the digestion of fat,

*__*protease*__ for the digestion of proteins,

*__*amylase*__ for the digestion of starches, and

*__*several other enzymes*__ which are for more specialized purposes.

Dr. Scott Anderson says that aging reduces the production of pancreatic enzymes, in addition to pancreatic diseases, which leads to incomplete digestion of food which, in turn, causes gas, bloating, and discomfort. Malnutrition and arthritis are related to the poor health of pancreas. Pancreas produces another enzyme known as ***elastase*** and when its levels drop it indicates that general deficiency of enzymes is affecting the digestion of sugars, fats, proteins, and starches. Reducing intake of sugars and starches, and taking supplements can relieve this problem. Bicarbonate produced by pancreas provides help to neutralize the stomach acids. Bicarbonate also neutralizes insulin which is directly released in to the blood to regulate sugar levels in the blood.

Pancreas has been called the precious pancreas, because its help to digest food through various enzymes crucial for the body. Extreme care should be provided to maintain pancreas in good health by minimizing consumption of starches and sugars in our daily food intake.

PANCREATIC CANCER

Pancreatic cancer is the 5th leading cancer in American women, and the number is increasing as the aging population grows each year. In pancreas two major glands secrete a variety of juices and hormones.

> **EXOCRINE GLANDS** secrete juices containing digestive enzymes which are passed in to the small intestine to breakdown carbohydrates, protein, and fat to help us digest the food we eat. More than 90% of all pancreatic cancer occurs in the ***exocrine cells*** which line the duct of pancreas.
>
> **ENDOCRINE GLANDS** secrete hormones like insulin, glucagons, somatostatin, and pancreatic polypeptide. Endocrine cells are clustered in groups throughout the pancreas and secrete hormones directly in to the bloodstream. The ***endocrine cell*** cancers are rare.

Most frequently, cancer develops at the head of the pancreas from where it can cause blockage of the common bile duct that connects the pancreas to the gallbladder and the liver. This blockage can prevent the bile from entering the small intestinc, and resulting in the disruption of the digestion process which will add to the problem by presenting an additional health problem: jaundice. About 40,000 Americans die of pancreatic cancer each year, which is very close to the number diagnosed.

Cancer of Pancreas

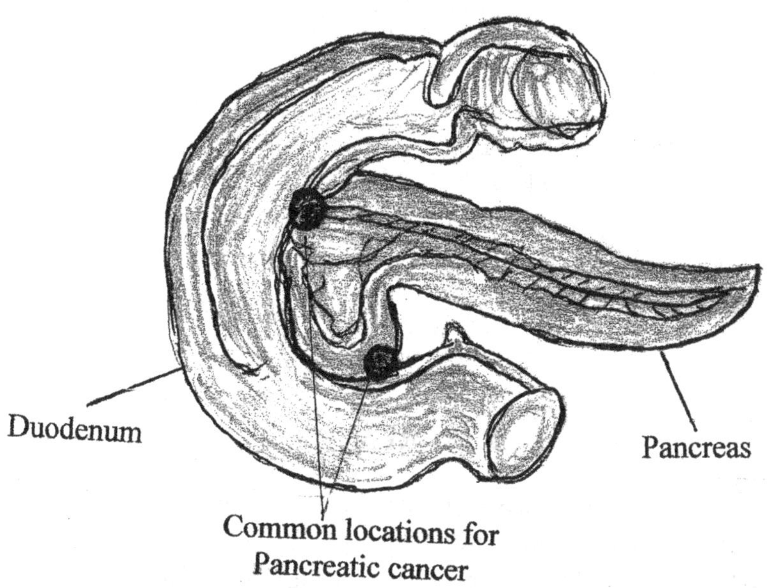

SUMPTOMS OF PANCREATIC CANCER

*Sustained abdominal pain which is mild and difficult to pinpoint.
*Pain traveling from the abdomen to the back.
*Poor appetite.
*Weight loss and weakness.
*Metallic taste in the mouth.
*Recurring blood clots in the leg.
*Gastro-intestinal bleeding.
*Vomiting and / or diarrhea.
*Jaundice.
*Fluid in the lining that covers the lungs.

CAUSES OF PANCREATIC CANCER

*Hereditary or genetic.

*Old age.
*Tobacco smoking
*Regular exposure to certain petroleum products and its fumes.
*Excessive dietary fat and excessive protein.
*Tobacco smoking puts women at risk which is three times that of non smokers.
*Diabetics are at a very high risk of getting pancreatic cancer.

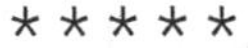

PANCREATITIS

Pancreatitis is best described as the acute inflammation of the pancreas. Pancreas gets inflamed when the excessive quantities of enzymes get build up inside due to the blockage of its ducts. Large quantities of stagnant enzymes within pancreas start breaking down its own tissue which starts the process of ***self digesting***, or auto digesting as described by Dr. Trent Nichols.

CAUSES

*Stones in the duct connecting pancreas to duodenum (the upper portion of the small intestine) and blocking the flow of digestive juices in to the intestine.
*Excessive alcohol consumption is the most prominent cause.
*Bacterial and viral infection inside of pancreas can cause inflammation.
*Damage to the blood vessels, hemorrhage, and other injuries.
*Inherited condition, or a genetic problem.

*Not fully formed ducts, and therefore can't function fully (birth defect).
*Scarring of pancreatic outlet causing inflammation, and resulting in obstruction
*Diabetes is more likely to cause gallstones due to chronic inflammation.
*High levels of calcium in the body.
*High levels of triglycerides in the body.
*Physical damage to pancreas caused by an accident.

RECOMMENDATIONS

*Stopping consumption of alcohol which has a strong link to gallstone formation.
*Eliminating fatty foods from your diet.
*Bringing down the triglycerides level in your blood.
*Drinking lots of clean water, that is, more than 8 glasses each day
*Taking enzymes in supplements.
*Adding hot peppers, garlic, onions, ginger, lemon, vinegar, pickles, and other spicy and sour condiments in your daily food intake.

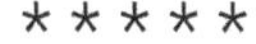

SKIN CANCER

Skin is the largest organ of the body measuring 16.1 sq ft to 21.5 sq ft, and containing about 1,000 nerve endings, 6,000 ***melanocytes*** (dark pigment ***melanin*** producing cells), more than 2 million sweat glands, and 20 blood vessels. It has multiple layers of epithelial tissues, and guards the underlying muscles, ligaments, bones, and the internal organs. It protects the body against excessive water loss, and pathogens. It provides insulation to the body, and regulates its temperature, maintains sensations, and produces chemicals that make vitamin D with the assistance of sunshine. Yet, about 35,000 skin cells die and are discarded each minute, and new cells replace them on a continuous basis. It is estimated that the top layer of our skin, ***epidermis***, is completely replaced in about a month, regularly.

Skin performs some additional very important tasks for the body. It contains DNA enzymes that help reverse the damage caused by ultra violet rays of the sun. People who lack these genes for the protective enzymes suffer skin cancer. Damaged skin will be healed by the skin itself by forming a scar tissue. Skin absorbs oxygen, nitrogen, and carbon dioxide. It is water resistant, so that the essential nutrients are not washed out. There are 3 layers of the skin.

> ***EPIDERMIS*** is the top layer, provides protection against water, and serves as a barrier to infections. There are no blood vessels in the skin; it is fed by dermis (the skin layer just below it). It contains ***keratinocytes*** (cells) which produce a protein, called ***keratin,*** which provides protection to the skin. Also, it contains ***melanocytes*** , the cells that produce melanin for the skin color, mostly at the lower level of epidermis. ***Langerhans***' are also found here, which work with the immune system to fight the invading foreign elements. At the lowest level ***merkel cells*** are found which are sensory receptors and provide sensory response to touch.
>
> ***DERMIS*** is the skin layer just below the epidermis, and is tightly connected to it. This second layer contains hair follicles, nerve endings, lymphatic nodes, blood vessels, sweat glands, etc.
>
> ***HYPODERMIS*** is not exactly a part of the skin, and lies just below the dermis. Its purpose and function is to attach the

skin to the underlying bones and muscles, and supply it with blood vessels and nerves.

MOST COMMON SKIN CANCERS

Almost all skin cancers originate in the outer layer of skin known as ***epidermis.*** All over the epidermis, there are ***melanocytes cells*** that produce a protective pigment called ***melanin.*** Cancer can start in heavily pigmented tissue such as a mole, as well as in the normally pigmented skin. There are more than 1,000,000 cases of the most common form of skin cancers occur in the United States, each year. By age 65, each of us will develop some form of cancer. There are three types of most common cancers: basal cell carcinoma, squamous cell carcinoma, and melanoma.

1-**Basal Cell Carcinoma** is the most common variety of cancer. It doesn't spread, and can be treated very easily. Most prominent symptoms include the appearance of bumps which are shiny and waxy on the face, ears, and neck; reddish brown patch on the chest or the back, or bleeding ulcer like oval bumps, etc.

2-**Squamous Cell Carcinoma** may appear on your sun-exposed skin. It can be treated easily. Unlike basal cell carcinoma, it is more likely to spread. The most visible signs to recognize this type of skin cancer are the appearance of a flat spot that becomes a bleeding sore that won't heal, a firm reddish wart like bump on the lips, face, neck, hands, and arms.

3- **Melanoma** is the most dangerous type of skin cancer which is responsible for most cancer deaths in the United States. It can appear anywhere on your body, although most commonly on the arms and legs. It can be treated successfully in early stages, however, if untreated it can spread to other parts and cause death. All women should inspect their body frequently and identify if there is an unusual change, appearance of spots, moles, etc. on the skin to determine if there are any signs of melanoma. If some unusual signs are visible then discuss with your doctor about the severity of this condition. Certain signs to look for are:

*shiny, firm, dome shaped bumps located anywhere on the body
*if a mole on your body is changing color and size, or if it bleeds
*a lesion with blue, red, white, blue-black spots on your trunk or limbs
*brownish or dark brown spots-- small or large-- with speckles on your body
*spot, blister, wound, scab, or injury on the palm, fingertips, toes, soles, mucous membrane lining of your mouth, nose, vagina, and anus.

This will provide you with some knowledge and the talking points during your visit to the doctor.

SYMPTOMS

*An inflamed or open skin wound which would not heal.
*A change in color of any highly pigmented spot or a mole on the skin.
*A flesh, colored and oval in shape, bump on the skin.
*A reddish brown or bluish black patch of skin on the chest or back.
*A flat dark brown or red spot with occasional bleeding remains unhealed.
*Mostly develops in areas exposed to the sun, lips, ear, skin, scalp, arms, legs, hands, etc.

*Can also develop beneath the finger nails, spaces between the toes, toenails, and genital area.
*Skin cancer affects all skin colors.
*Dark skinned women may develop melanoma on the covered areas of their body, instead of the exposed skin.
*A cluster of dark, shiny, and firm bumps on the skin.

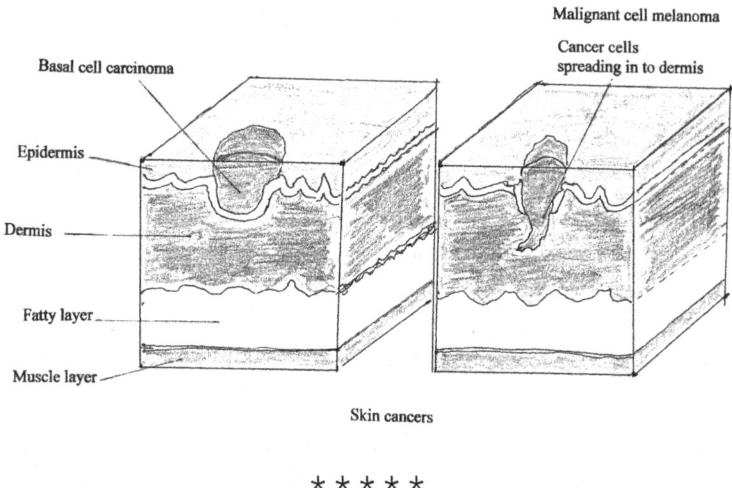

Skin cancers

* * * * *

LESS COMMON SKIN CANCERS

All cancers should be considered dangerous disregarding the degree of their overall impact on the population. Often, less common cancers and other less common diseases are hard to cure because relatively less research has been developed.

Kaposi Sarcoma is a serious type of skin cancer which develops in the blood vessels of dermis which is the second layer of the skin, and causes red or purple patches on the skin or the mucous membranes. It mostly occurs due to the weakened immune system of the body. Women who have AIDS and their immune system is down are generally the victims of Kaposi Sarcoma. Also, women who have undergone organ transplant and have weakened immune system can get this type of cancer.

Merkel Cell Carcinoma is a rare type of cancer. It develops in the second layer of the skin in the hair follicles. Red, pink, or blue nodules, up to 2 inch in length appear on the sun-exposed area of legs, arms, neck, and the head. It has tendency to grow rapidly, and the capability to spread to other parts of the body.

Sebaceous Gland Carcinoma is an aggressive type of cancer, though its occurrence is not so common. It originates in the oil glands of the skin. It can develop anywhere on the body, however, mostly on the eyelids. It is hard and painless nodule.

CAUSES & RISK FACTORS

Skin cancer begins in the skin's top layer called epidermis. It provides a protective layer of skin cells that your body continually sheds. Here are the main types of cells in the top layer of the skin (epidermis): The ***Squamous Cells*** lie just below the skin surface. They are the skin's inner lining. The ***Basal Cells*** are located just beneath the squamous cells, and produce new skin cells. The ***Melanocytes*** are located in the lower part of the top layer of the skin (epidermis), and produce melanin the pigment that gives the skin its normal color. More melanin is produced by the skin when you are in the sun to protect the deeper layers of your skin. Repeated exposure to the sun stimulates production of melanin, which is why the tanned skin becomes darker in color. Under normal conditions, the healthy new cells push the older cells upward to the skin surface where they die and eventually pushed out. This process is controlled by the DNA that contains the instructions for every biological and chemical process in the body. Skin cancer occurs when this process is not functioning properly.

A lot of changes in the instructions occur when the DNA gets damaged, which can cause new cells to grow out of control and form a cluster of cancer cells.

*__How the DNA in the cells gets damaged?__ ***Ultra Violet (UV)*** light from the sun or the sunlamp can damage the DNA. Wave lengths of ultra violet rays are very short and lie between the wave lengths of visible light and the x-rays (shorter than 4000 angstrom). Reflected light from water, sand, and snow is equally intense as sunlight. Ultra violet rays have been divided in to 3 categories: UV-A, UV-B, and UV-C, out of which only UV-A and UV-B reach the earth; UV-C is absorbed by the ozone.

UV-B is harmful and can change the DNA of the skin cell. UV-B can turn on or activate ***oncogene*** which can turn a normal cell in to a malignant cell. UV-B rays are responsible for sunburns and many basal cell and squamous cell cancers. ***UV-A*** penetrates the skin more deeply than UV-B, and weakens the skin's immune system, and increases the risk of melanoma. Tanning parlors who provide the services of tanning use high doses of UV-A on their clients to give them quick tanning. Obviously, it is very dangerous for the skin, and cancer causing.

*__Fair skinned__ women are more likely to get skin cancer because they have lower quantities of pigment (melanin) in their skin to protect them.

*__History of sunburns__ is an important indicator of your getting skin cancer. If you have had blistering sunburns as a child and as a young woman then you are more likely to develop skin cancer.

*__Radiation treatment, x-rays, and scans__ can cause skin cancer, though the symptoms may not appear immediately.

*__Excessive sun exposure__ increases your risk of getting skin cancer. To start with, a tan is your skin's injury response to an excessive exposure to ultra-violet radiation.

*__High altitude locations__ have very strong sunlight because of the clean and clutter free atmosphere at that height, and the inhabitants are at high risk of developing skin cancer, just like the habitants of warm and sunny areas where plenty of exposure to ultra violet radiation occurs.

*__Having skin injuries__ that don't seem to heal completely, known as ***actinic keratosis***, is a dangerous sign of its developing in to a skin cancer. These are dehydrated patches of brown or dark pink color appear on the face, hands, and arms of fair skinned women whose skin has been damaged by the sun's ultra violet rays.

*__Personal history of skin cancer__ tells a different story. If you have had skin cancer before and you completely healed from it, it will return once again. Even basal cell and squamous cell carcinoma that was successfully removed from your skin will return on the same spot after about 3 years.

*Women with **HIV/AIDS** or **leukemia**, and those who are taking immune suppressant drugs after the organ transplant have weakened immune system. Such women and others who have weakened immune system are at a high risk of getting skin cancer.

*Women with **fragile skin** that has been injured, damaged, or weakened by other skin conditions are more susceptible to skin cancer. Certain medication for psoriasis and eczema may increase your risk of getting skin cancer, according to Mayo clinic.

*Exposure to **environmental hazards** like: pesticides, herbicides, and a variety of industrial chemicals can increase the risk of skin cancer.

*The risk of developing skin cancer is increased with **age**. Damage to the skin inflicted during childhood may not become apparent until middle age, because skin cancer develops slowly. However, basal cell carcinoma and squamous cell carcinoma are increasing in women as young as 40 years.

RECOMMENDATIONS

*Avoid intense sun exposure by staying out of it during a good portion of late morning and afternoon when sun's rays are most intense. Follow the Eastern women who often take out their umbrellas during the mid day sun exposure,

*When outside in the sun, wear long sleeve shirts, pants, hat, UV blocking sunglasses, and if culture allows use an umbrella.

*Take vitamin-B which contains PABA which is used in sun screen lotions.

*Check your body regularly for any moles, bumps, red or dark spots, rashes, etc about which consult your doctor without delay, especially if you have a family history of melanoma.

*Before using any lotions, sunscreens, or medication discuss with your doctor.

*Avoid visiting skin tanning parlors.

*Stop using suntan lamps immediately, unless they have been proven safe and recommended by your doctor.

*Try your best to keep your skin moist and healthy by making sure that it does not get dried out, because dried out skin cracks and allows bacteria, foreign elements, and toxins to enter thereby causing a host of health problems besides causing blemishes.

*Drink a lot of water every day, that is, more than 8 glasses.

*Oil massage should be a part of every woman's lifestyle on a weekly basis.

*For healthy skin, take, omega-3 containing fish oil, flaxseed oil, fruits, vegetables, some milk products.

*For facial, try using paste made out of cucumber peel, small wedges of orange and lemon with the peel, a little whole milk, and a small quantity of egg white. Keep this paste on your face for a couple of hours or longer. Large quantities of paste can be made and stored in the refrigerator for regular applications.

*Get involved in light physical activities that cause sweating. More than 2 million sweat glands in the skin need to be activated to cleanse the body. If possible stay away from air conditioned and highly heated environment, thereby allowing the skin to secrete sweat naturally. Sweat cleanse the body, moistens, and lubricates the skin.

*Minimize your exposure to x-rays, MRI, and other forms of scanning, because their waves can damage the DNA and the cells in your body.

*If under Radiation Therapy then request for lower intensity and fewer doses.

* * * * * *

STOMACH CANCER

Stomach cancer is most common in women over 50 years of age. It usually produces no unique symptoms other than some indigestion, loss of weight, loss of some appetite, etc.

SYMPTOMS

*A bloated or full feeling, loss of appetite.
*Indigestion, heartburn.
*Discomfort while eating.
*Stomach pain.
*Experiencing a feeling of nausea, or vomiting after meals.
*Constipation or diarrhea.
*Blood in the stool, or dark patches.
*Coughing blood, or vomiting blood.

Often cancer develops on the stomach's glandular lining, although it can form anywhere in the stomach. There are other two prominent locations where it can develop, that are, right below the ***junction of esophagus and stomach***, and the other is where stomach meets the upper portion of small intestine, called ***duodenum***.

Unless treated immediately, it can spread to other parts of the body, which can increase the risk for the patient by tenfold. Women with surgically removed tumor in the stomach have less than 20% survival rate within a period of 5 years after surgery.

Cancer can form at the site of an ulcer, or an ***ulcer*** can become cancerous. Women who consume salted, smoked, pickled, and barbecued animal foods, which contain nitrites and other carcinogens, are more at risk of developing stomach cancer. The stomach cancer is also caused by ***aflatoxins***, a toxin, produced by a fungus known as ***aspergillus flavus*** found in stored nuts, corn, seeds, and some other dried products, for a long time under humid environment, and can cause ***aflatoxicosis*** (poisoning by aflatoxins) which is often fatal. Women who smoke and drink have higher risk of developing stomach cancer than who don't.

Ulcers, which could become the ground for developing a cancer, develop in the stomach, duodenum, and at the bottom of esophagus, primarily start from excessive stress levels, genetic predisposition, alcohol abuse, over indulgence in rich foods, caffeine, tobacco, etc thereby increasing the acid levels of the stomach. High acid levels erode away the lining of the stomach, duodenum, and esophagus. Other contributors to stomach ulcers are over use of aspirin, ibuprofen, naproxen, and infection by ***helicobacter pylori***. Increasing number of researchers believe that the primary cause of developing a peptic ulcer is due to the infection of helicobacter pylori.

On worldwide basis, chronic ulcers, stomach irritation, anemia, and gastritis are also linked to stomach cancer. Women workers who inhale carcinogen fumes and dust emanating at workplace, especially coal mines, metal refineries, etc, are susceptible to getting stomach cancer.

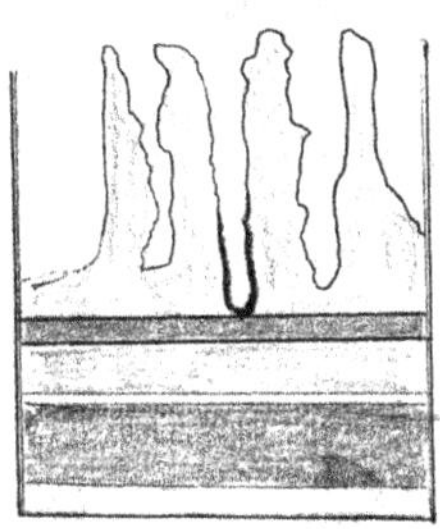

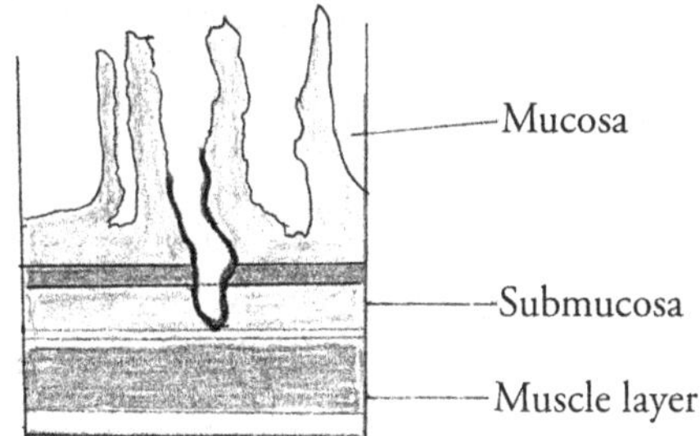

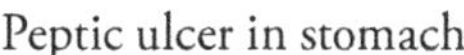

Peptic ulcer in stomach

Progressed ulcer penetrating muscle layer

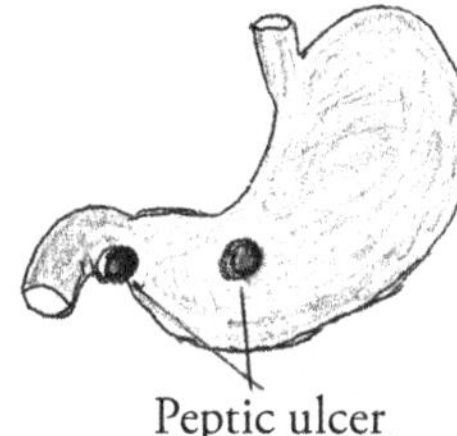

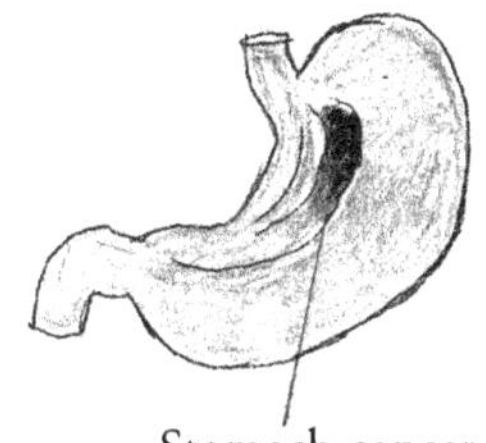

RECOMMENDATIONS

*Stop eating pickled, barbecued, smoked, and salted animal foods.

*Eat as many green and leafy vegetables and fruits as you can.

*Eat garlic regularly with the main meals of the day, preferably raw.

*Give up smoking, and consumption of alcohol.

*Stop using over the counter medicines like aspirin, ibuprofen, naproxen…..

*Live and breathe in an environment free of dust, toxins, smoke, industrial fumes, etc.

*Move away from industrial and automobile traffic environments.

*Regularly consult with your doctor.

*Minimize levels of stress by being involved in some kind of activity.
*Maintain regular sleeping and resting hours.

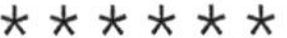

CANCER IN LOWER BODY

CERVICAL CANCER

Cervix is the neck of the women's uterus located just above the vagina. 90% of the cervical cancers originate in the surface cells lining the cervix. Cervix cancer is more common in women who have borne children. In some women healthy cells enter an abnormal phase called ***dysphasia***. In the initial stage these cells are not cancerous, but they may become. If and when they become cancerous, they can invade the lining of the cervix, spread to other tissues, or enter in to the blood stream and travel to other parts of the body. Each year, about 60,000 American women between the ages 40 and 60 experience cervical cancers.

SYMPTOMS

*Pain and/or difficulty in urinating.
*Blood in urine.
*Vaginal bleeding between menstrual periods.
*Bleeding from the rectum after passing stool, diarrhea.
*In some women vaginal bleeding may occur after entering in to menopause.

*Menstruation may be very heavy and lasting abnormally longer time.
*Bloody or watery discharge from vagina, often heavy and foul smelling.
*Swelling in the legs.
*Loss of weight, tiredness, loss of appetite.

CAUSES & RISK FACTORS

*85% of cervical cancer cases are linked to sexually transmitted infections. ***Genital herpes*** and several ***human papilloma viruses*** (HPV) which cause genital warts are linked to the cervical cancer.

*Make-up of genes is also a dominant factor in developing cervical cancer.

*Cervical cancer is more common in women who smoke tobacco.

*Women with weakened immune system due to various experiences of infections, ailments, diseases, etc are susceptible to cervical cancer.

*Women who are obese, take birth control pills, and/or are alcohol abusers will have increased risk of cervical cancer.

RECOMMENDATIONS

*Women who are sexually active should talk to their doctor about Pap smear and Pelvic exam.
*Protect yourself from sexually transmitted diseases with doctor recommended measures including condoms.

*Consult your doctor about safe birth control measures.

*Raise your self esteem to a much higher level, and learn to practice abstinence.
*Maintain healthy body weight levels.
*Maintain consumption of alcohol to maximum one drink per day.
*Give up smoking.

OTHER CERVICAL CONDITIONS

Cervicitis** is a condition of acute and chronic inflammation of the cervix. The symptoms are grayish or whitish vaginal discharge abnormally, pain during sexual activity, and backache. It is generally caused by sexually transmitted diseases like ***genital herpes, ***chlamydia, trychomoniasis***, and ***gonorrhea***.

***Cervical eversion** occurs when the red columnar cells, lining the inner cervical canal, begin to form on the outer vaginal part of the cervix. Women who are pregnant or are on birth control pills experience this condition the most.

***Cervical erosion** occurs when the pink squamous cell tissue of the cervix has been worn away and the red exposed sores on the surface are exposed. This condition may cause bloody vaginal discharge.

Cervix stenosis** is partial or total narrowing of the cervix and forming an obstruction, usually caused by infection, polyps, uterine fibroids; and ***Cervical incompetence which causes premature opening of cervix during pregnancy, which can cause miscarriage.

***Cervical cysts** and **Cervical polyps** are generally non cancerous, though, require removal by surgery, because they can affect fertility.

*__Genital warts__ are caused by ***human papilloma virus*** and there are many types of this virus which can cause cervical cancer.

*__Dysphasia__ is another problematic condition in the cervix which, in essence, is the abnormal development of cervical cells, and is a precancerous condition.

RECOMMENDATIONS

*Use condoms, diaphragms, cervical caps when having sex.
*Abstinence is better than sexual activity; frequent exposure to semen brings women closer to having dysphasia in their cervix.
*Eat a lot of green vegetables, fruits, and nuts to improve your immune system to ward of ***cervicitis*** (inflammation of cervix) and many other diseases.
*Have your cervix screened from time to time to make sure there is no inflammation or erosion in the cervix, because it can cause infertility.
*Stop smoking tobacco because it causes many kinds of cancers in the body, including cervical cancer.

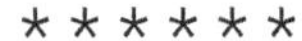

COLORECTAL CANCER

Cancer of the colon and the rectum are the most prevalent cancers in the western world. It is a slow growing disease, and the symptoms appear much later when the damage has already been done. Typical symptoms of Colorectal Cancer are bleeding, fatigue, and pain from the colon and the rectum. This type of cancer develops from the cells of layers that line the inner walls of the intestinal tract, known as ***Epithelial Layer.*** About 700,000 colorectal cancer deaths occur each year through out the world.

SYMPTOMS

In general, the symptoms are common with several other serious health conditions; however, medical checkups should be made immediately after noticing frequent attacks of

*Nausea
*Heartburn and indigestion particularly after meals
*Loss of appetite and loss of weight
*Ribbon like thin stools
*Some blood with in stools,
*Fatigue
*Pain in the lower portion of the large intestine and the rectum
*Changes in the bowel movements
*Persistent constipation, diarrhea, gas pains
*Stomach pain, bloating, etc.

Colorectal Cancer is closely related to various other types of serious health conditions like: colitis, Crohn's disease, cancer of breasts, cancer of ovaries, cancer of pancreas, and intestinal polyps. The risk of getting a Colorectal Cancer is 20 times higher if a woman has ulcerative colitis. Researchers have established that the occurrence of Colorectal Cancer will be experienced by those with the family history, and those with specific personal habits in accompaniment with the environmental factors. Scientists have identified a particular gene for hereditary nonpolyposis colorectal cancer which is said to predispose women to colorectal cancer and cancers of uterine, stomach, intestinal, and other organs.

Tumors start as polyps on the intestinal wall of rectum or colon. Over time they grow to become cancer causing tumors, and in time they penetrate the intestinal wall of the colon or rectum. Once inside the wall of colon or rectum, they can travel to other parts of the body and spread cancer.

Colorectal cancer

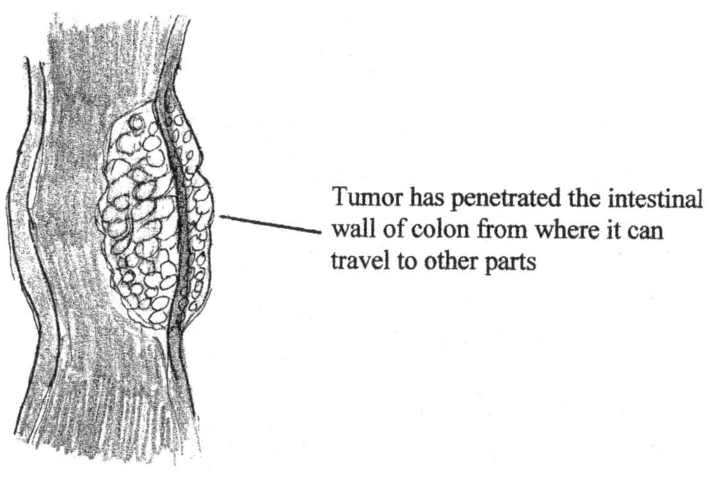

CAUSES

Some researchers believe that Colorectal Cancer is caused by fats of all kinds, while other link it to the methodology of cooking all of our foods, yet some other think that it is mostly environmental, and most think genetics play the most important role in casting the destiny of the patient. No matter how the picture is perceived, there are fatalities and exceptions. During this time when cancer research is still in full swing to determine the proximate cause or causes of Colorectal Cancer, we should focus on the risk reducing methods to offset this disease in women.

RECOMMENDATIONS

To lower the probability of getting Colorectal Cancer, I will list a few suggestions which are simple and make sense in women's everyday life.

*By increasing the ***non-soluble fiber*** in your daily diet will increase the transit time of your food traveling from the mouth to the anus. Women at home can easily manage the regular intake of sufficient quantities of fiber in their diet. Women who are working outside in the field or offices may not get enough fiber in the foods eaten at the restaurants or coffee shops and, therefore, should resort to taking fiber pills with plenty of water to overcome this deficiency. Bowel movement should be at least once day, though twice a day is even better.

****Fatty acids*** protect the lining of the stomach and the intestinal tract, and the grain fiber becomes a big catalyst to promote the utilization of fatty acids. ***Phytic acid***, found in the grains, is of clear or pale yellow water soluble liquid usually used to chelate heavy metals, in the manufacture of animal fats, vegetable oils, and also as a water softening agent. ***Phytic acid*** is believed to play an important role in the prevention of Colon Cancer.

****Selenium*** is generally essential for our body. It is an important antioxidant which protects cells and tissues from the free radicals in women's body. Also, it enhances the levels of ***Glutathione Peroxidase***, an essential enzyme which protects the gut from getting cancer. It protects women's immune system, intestines, and may prevent cancer, stroke, heart disease, and arthritis. Women with advanced stages of cancer may show lower levels of selenium. The prominent sources of selenium are bananas, kiwi, strawberries, oranges; apples, etc.

Animal fat** contains higher level of saturated fat which is closely associated with Colorectal Cancer and should be minimized in food intake, if not eliminated altogether. ***Fish oil, on the other hand, is a beneficial fat. People living on the islands and the coastal areas throughout the world seldom experience an incidence of Colorectal Cancer. The cooking oil used in cooking the animal foods may also be a player in this type of cancer.

Hetero cyclic amines** appear when meat is fried or barbecued on high temperatures. Some people like the meat to be smoky, dark brown, almost burnt, and sizzling before eating it, and inadvertently they expose themselves to ***hetero cyclic amines (HCA) which cause alterations in the genetic materials, and are carcinogens. PhIP is the most cancer causing substance in HCA, and is found in barbecued and fried foods. HCA can cause Colorectal Cancer. Stewed or baked (un-burnt) meats don't show presence of HCA. Also, HCA is not found in vegetables. Therefore avoiding fried and barbecued meats will reduce the colorectal cancer risk, and increasing the intake of vegetable source diet will bring intestinal health and possibly eliminate the occurrence of cancer in women.

Casein** is a protein precipitated from milk, which form the basis of cheese and some plastics. Casein is found in a concentrated form in cooked milk containing foods that have been cooked or prepared at high temperatures. It is harder to digest. It has been linked to the uncontrolled growth of intestinal tissue. Women who find it impossible to eliminate pizza, whole milk, creams, etc. from their diet may choose to minimize consumption of these foods for the sake of maintaining healthy intestinal walls. On the other hand, according to Dr. Jonathan Wright, ***sphingolipids are found in fat free milk, which tend to protect the inside of intestinal walls and reduce the risk of getting Colorectal Cancer.

****Polyps*** and cancer emerge from the epithelial layer of the intestinal tract. Western diet produces an excess number of epithelial cells in the intestinal tract thereby increasing the risk of polyp growth and colon cancer. Taking calcium and vitamin D supplements with meals may prevent this risk. Calcium binds itself to the irritating fatty acids and inactivates them, which reduces the risk of colon cancer. Also, vitamin D and its breakdown product ***'metabolite'*** can reduce the risk of colorectal cancer. Also, thiamine, folic acid, and vitamin B-6 act as protective agents against Colorectal Cancer. Women with family history of Colorectal Cancer should take extra care in taking the proper supplements, diet, and precautionary measures, because they are pre-disposed to this disease through genes.

****The friendly bacteria*** in the intestinal tract should be maintained healthy, and should never be allowed to get altered or mutated. A healthy colony of beneficial bacteria in the gut is healthy for the body. The friendly bacteria thrive on diet which contains adequate fiber. To maintain the health and population of beneficial bacteria, women should consume cultured products like yogurt and fermented products like pickles, pickled vegetables, sauerkraut, etc along with other fiber containing foods. The family of bacteria known as ***clostridium*** is toxic to intestinal lining, and is linked to the Colorectal Cancer. Intake of cultured and fermented foods does not allow clostridium to grow and thrive. Women should develop a habit of consuming at least one cup of yogurt every day, and some pickles as condiments with each meal.

****Alcohol consumption and tobacco smoking*** can lead to high intestinal toxicity, damage the liver, damage the intestinal lining and allow the foreign substances and free radicals to enter and colonize where detection and medication become ineffective. Similarly tobacco smoking provides the smoker about 4,000 compounds of chemicals which cause heart attacks, stroke, cancer, etc. There are about 400 carbon compounds in tobacco smoking that are lethal to humans, beside a variety of toxins, metals, tar, etc. which cause stroke, heart disease, lung cancer, cancer of various organs including colorectal cancer. Stopping to smoke, avoiding smoke environment, and stopping to drink alcohol should be the first step taken by all women at risk of Colorectal or any other kind of cancer.

*Today, most women are working, or want to work and be financially independent. ***Occupational health hazards*** are always there for which only personal awareness and care will gain any mileage. Employers would go only so far in protecting your health, that is, within the legal requirements, while the total responsibility rests with you. Researchers have learned that asbestos, certain chemicals, cements, and several other substances are linked to the right side of the colon. There are metals, toxins, chemicals, and poisons in the water, air, foods, kitchenware; etc which put an enormous burden on our physiology, and therefore each protective step improves our well being.

Unattended Colorectal Cancer tends to grow rapidly and eventually cause death. Grains, vegetables, fruits, legumes, nuts, nutritional supplements, fermented foods, cultured foods, etc. help us nourish our body in a non-cancer causing way. Some women have been given to understand that radiation, chemotherapy, surgery, and medication will solve any and every problem. Please don't depend upon it; instead it should be the last option of any woman. The first option should be self health management, so cancer never appears.

* * * * * *

URINARY BLADDER CANCER

Bladder is an organ located in the lower abdomen, just below the womb (uterus). It is like a hollow balloon to store urine produced by kidneys. Urethra is a flexible tube connected to the lower part of the bladder from which the urine passes to the exit point. Bladder has an outer layer of muscles, which squeezes the bladder cavity to push the urine through the urethra tube for discharging the accumulated urine out of the body. There are several layers of bladder's outer wall. Listing from the inside of the bladder to the outside, these layers are:

*Epithelium
*Lamina propria
*Mucos and submucosa
*Superficial muscle
*Deep muscle

TYPES OF BLADDER CANCER

****Transitional Cell Cancer*** is possibly the earliest stage of bladder cancer, which is present strictly on the surface and, most cases, has not penetrated the inner layers of the bladder wall. Most of the reported cancer cases fall in to this category, that is, 90% of about 75,000 cases per years.

****Squamous Cell Cancer*** is an invasive cancer. Its appearance is flat and thin. It resembles to skin cancer, and is primarily caused by a parasite known as ***schistosoma,*** which can enter the human body by penetrating the skin.

****Adenocarcinoma*** is a tumor which resembles in appearance to the tumors of gland forming cells in the intestinal tract. According to Dr. Derek Raghavan of *Cleveland Clinic*, Adenocarinoma, an intrusive cancer, may occur in the urachus, a remnant of a fetal structure that connects the bladder to the umbilicus before birth.

***Small Cell Anaplastic** bladder cancer is similar to the small cell cancer usually found in the lung. This rapidly growing cancer is found on the bladder wall and in other organs, and is suspected of playing a role in cellular growth control.

Choriocarcinoma** and ***Sarcoma are two rare types of bladder cancers which are found on the muscle layers of the bladder.

The physicians will stage and grade your bladder cancer, if you have one. It is helpful to know the process briefly, so that you understand what the doctor is talking about and what should be asked in response. The process is just to determine how deep the cancer has penetrated in the bladder lining and the bladder muscle, or beyond. There are categories of severity of this type of cancer, which are:
T-a…affected area is the epithelium
T-1…affected area is the lamina propria
T-2a. affected area is the superficial muscle
T-2b..affected area is the deep muscle
T-3a..affected area is the adjacent tissue
T-3b.affected area is the adjacent fat or the peritoneum
T-4a.affected area is the adjacent organ-vagina or uterus, (prostate in men).

SYMPTOMS

*Blood in the urine with or without pain. It is also called ***hematuria.*** 85% of patients with bladder cancer have blood

in their urine. The presence of blood in the urine may appear and disappear at times. Visit to the doctor and blood test are the only ways to determine if there is blood, especially after you have seen it once.
*Pain or burning sensation
*Feeling to urinate when there is no urine to discharge
*Getting up frequently during the night to urinate.
*Backache, abdominal pain, fatigue, and weight loss may be additional symptoms

Bladder cancer is the 10th most common cancer among women. Most commonly, it occurs in women in the ages of 50 and 70. Caucasian women are most susceptible to bladder cancer.

CAUSES & RISK FACTORS

*Tobacco smoke, first hand or second hand, is a major cause of bladder cancer. 80% of bladder cancer is believed to be caused by tobacco smoke.

*A parasite known as ***schistosomia*** is linked to a type of bladder cancer called **Squamous Cell Carcinoma. *Schistosomia***, most commonly found in the middle Eastern countries, Far East, Africa, Caribbean, and South America. It is mostly found in fresh water from where it gets on human skin and thereafter it travels to various organs. About 100.000.000 people get it worldwide.

*Working in
-textile, dyes, rubber, and chemical industries
-some pharmaceutical and pesticide manufacturing environment
-coal and gas industries
-aluminum, iron, and steel industries

*Painters, hairdressers, truck drivers
*Sewage workers
*Women who had Pelvic Radiation treatment for cervical cancer
*Women who had chemotherapy with drugs like Cyclophosphamide or Ifosfamide.
*Inheritance of genes from parents.

RECOMMENDATIONS

*Avoid exposure to chemicals, auto fumes, industrial environment, toxic environment, and other hazardous industrial and polluted environments.
*Cover your head and body with clothing if you are working in toxic environment
*Wear hand gloves during working hours.
*Wear face masks wherever it is allowed or provided by the employer.
*Take a shower and clean your body on returning from polluted work environment each day.

*Increase the amount of fresh water, other liquids, and fresh vegetables and fruits intake during working hours.
*Minimize or eliminate solid foods, manufactured foods, breads, meats, etc. during working hours.
*Stop smoking tobacco and avoid smoke environment.
*Develop an option to move away from industrial zone.
*Develop an option to take up other source of making a living.
*Cleanse your body from the inside and outside regularly.
*Move to a clean environment.

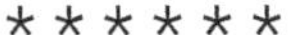

UTERINE CANCER (ENDOMETRIOSIS)

Uterine cancer or endometriosis is among the most common cancers in American women. It begins in the lining of uterus, called ***endometrium***. This lining or endometrium has special cells which have direct relationship with the cyclical hormonal changes. This lining is enriched with blood just before the menstrual cycle begins. Here, the nature is playing an important part by providing a nutritional environment for the fertilized egg to develop in to a baby. If the egg gets fertilized then there is sufficient supply of nutrition for it to develop in to a baby. If the egg is fertilized, no menstruation will occur. If there is no contact between egg and sperm then all that nutrition in the form of blood will be released. This release of blood from the uterus lining (endometrium) is called ***menstruation*** which occurs in almost all women every month.

In some women, the uterus lining tissues break away and travel to other areas like: vaginal vault, ovaries, etc. For some reason, these break away cells never lose their programmed behavior, and behave exactly in the same manner while in those foreign locations. Monthly hormonal changes affect them in the same manner as before when they were in the uterus lining. Responding to the monthly hormonal changes from a foreign location causes bleeding, swelling, and shrinking causing unbearable pain, primarily because blood cannot escape and it ends up irritating and scarring the surrounding tissue. This phenomenon is known as ***endometriosis.*** This condition makes it difficult for woman to get pregnant.

ENDOMETRIAL OR UTERINE CANCER

Uterine cancer is caused when the cells become abnormal and get out of body's normal rhythm. Abnormal cells grow out of balance and start dividing endlessly even when there is no need for them.

Normal and healthy cells grow and divide themselves in an orderly manner to maintain the body's normal function. This abnormal overgrowth destroys nearby tissues. These abnormal cells can travel and start growing in other parts of the body with a similar outcome of destruction of tissues. Endometrial cancer develops in the lining (endometrium) of the uterus due to overgrowth of cells which mutate and become cancer cells. The ovaries produce two hormones: e***strogen*** and ***progesterone***, and the balance between these hormones changes each month. When the balance shifts toward more estrogen which stimulates growth of endometrium, the risk of developing Endometrial Cancer is increased.

CAUSES & RISK FACTORS

*Too much exposure to estrogen stimulates the cell division and growth which has high chance of mutation to become cancer cells. Women who started menstruating early, their endometrium have been exposed to estrogen for a long time which puts them at additional risk of getting endometrial cancer.

*Women without pregnancy are at a high risk of getting endometrial cancer. Pregnancies decrease the chances of getting endometrial cancer in a woman, because estrogen and progesterone are produced, and progesterone offsets the risk factors related to estrogen.

*High fat diet has been linked to obesity and endometrial cancer, because it is directly linked to the estrogen production.

*Normally ovaries produce estrogen, but fat tissues can also produce estrogen. *American Cancer Society* says that over weight women have twice the risk, and obese women have three times of getting endometrial cancer.

*Diabetic women are at increased risk of getting endometrial cancer.

*Women above 55 have higher risk.

*Women with ovarian tumors are at higher risk.

*Failure to ovulate increases the lifetime exposure to estrogen, thereby increases the cancer risk.

*Women with history of breast cancer, ovarian cancers, etc are at higher risk.

*If your breast cancer was treated with tamoxifen, you have a higher risk, according to Mayo Clinic.

*White women are more likely candidates for endometrial cancer than black.

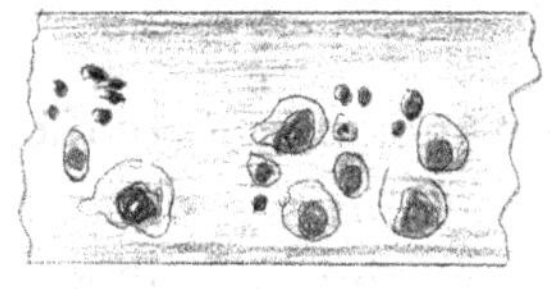

Endometriosis in vaginal lining

Runaway tissues respond to hormones by bleeding during menstruration

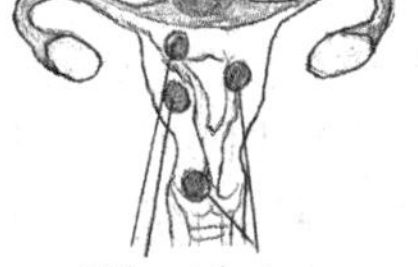

Fibroids in uterus

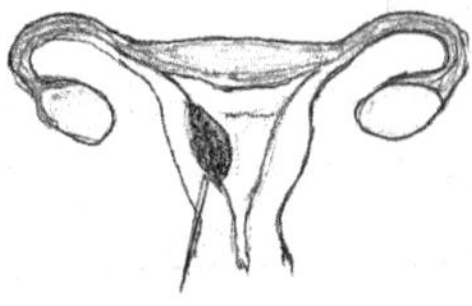

Uterine cancer

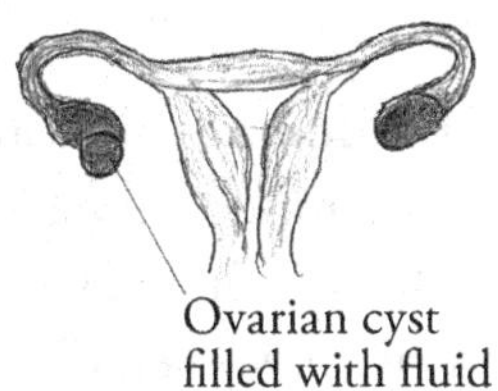

Ovarian cyst filled with fluid

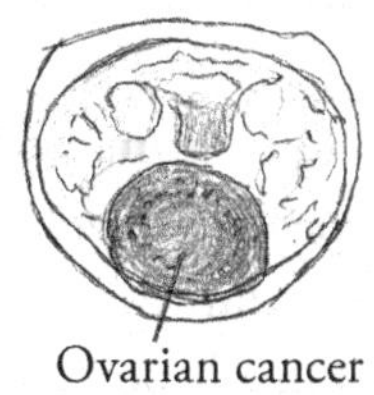

Ovarian cancer

RECOMMENDATIONS

*Take Pap smear and pelvic exam annually.
*If taking birth control pills then do consult your doctor about the pros and cons of it.
*Low fat and high fiber diet should be on your daily menu.
*Strict control of your weight must be practiced.

*Have regular check ups, and consultations with your physician.
*Vitamins A, C, and E containing fruits and vegetables should be plentiful in your diet.
*Take rest frequently throughout the day.
*Drink more than 8 glasses of clean water.

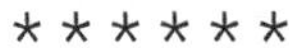

VAGINAL CANCER

Cancer of vagina is a disease in which malignant cancer cells form in the vagina. Vagina is the canal which starts from the cervix (the opening of the uterus) to the vaginal opening outside of the body. When a baby is born, it passes out through the vagina, also known as the birth canal. The vagina is self cleaning, and allows the secretions to flow downward, flushing out the dead cells and other substances. Normally, a vaginal discharge is clear or white in color. Cancer of vagina is different from the cancers of cervix and uterus. Following are the most prominent vaginal cancers:

*__Squamous cell carcinoma__ is the cancer that forms in the ***squamous cells*** in the lining of vagina. These cancer cells, flat and thin, grow slowly but can spread to the liver and the lungs. It occurs mostly in women of 60 or older.

*__Vaginal melanoma__ is the cancer which begins in the

melanocytes, the pigment producing cells in the lining of the vagina

Adenocarcinoma** is the cancer that originates in the ***glandular cells of the lining of vagina. Glandular cells make and release fluids such as mucus, and the cancer originating from it is more likely to spread to lungs and lymph nodes. It mostly occurs in women of age 30 or younger.

SYMPTOMS

*Bleeding or discharge, not related to menstruation.
*Pain during sexual intercourse.
*Lump in the vagina.
*Painful urination.
*Watery vaginal discharge with occasional foul smell.
*Unexplained constipation.

RISK FACTORS

*Women with vaginal intra-epithelial neoplasm (abnormal growth of new tissues) have high risk of vaginal cancer.
*Most women patients are 60 or older.
*Women who have been exposed to miscarriage prevention drug (DES) while in the womb (DES is given to pregnant women to prevent miscarriage).

*Women who have human papilloma virus (HPV), a sexually transmitted disease, are at high risk of getting vaginal cancer.
*Women with a history of gynecological cancer are at high risk.
*Women who have multiple sexual partners are at high risk.
*Women who started having sexual intercourse at a very early age are at risk.

*HIV infected women are at high risk.
*Tobacco smoking women are at high risk.

RECOMMENDATIONS

*Live a clean and orderly life.
*Have only one sexual partner, preferably your husband.
*Develop your immune system through healthy diet and lifestyle.
*Consult your personal physician regularly.
*Give up tobacco smoking, alcohol, fried foods, fats, sugars, and polluted environment.
*Seek alternative medications and therapies.

STROKE

Historically, people have associated Stroke condition with males only, probably because most of the time males complained, and got attended to. The ones who knew something about it had little or no knowledge about its causes, let alone its cure. Females were never considered as candidates for such health condition, even though they experienced a variety of stress levels; in many cases even higher than males. Somehow for unspecified reasons, the medical community ignored them even though death rate for women from stroke is at least equal to men, if not higher. Unattended stroke patients can die slowly, and women have died slowly of Stroke over thousands of years. The cause of their death remained unknown, or kept confidential for cultural or religious reasons, or labeled as female disease.

According to Center for Disease Control Center, Stroke is the third leading cause of death after Heart disease and cancer. Stroke is the leading cause of long term disability. We cannot ignore these facts. Also, we cannot ignore the fact that proportionately women suffer from Cardio Vascular Disease more than men.

Over the years several studies showed that of all the deaths caused by stroke 61% of them were women. These numbers demonstrate how little attention women have received over the years. Women were considered second class citizens, especially in response to their healthcare needs.

Each year, about 700,000 men and women suffer a Stroke out of which 500,000 are the first timers, and 200,000 are second or third or fourth. Each year Medicare spends billions of dollars on Stroke Survivors after they leave hospitals. Now, who can question the importance of Stroke incidence in the USA, and its subsequent impact on the survivors and the loved-ones.

U.S. Government has become increasingly aware of the toll caused by the incidence of Stroke in America, its cost, the resultant disability, and the yearly productive man-hours lost due to this debilitating and deadly health condition. According to Center for Disease Control (CDC)

> *Stroke is the third leading cause of death in America
> *more than 100 deaths occur from stroke every hour
> *One in four adults has some form of Cardio Vascular Disease (CVD)
> *Stroke is the leading cause of Disability
> *many survivors never recover
> *20% of Stroke victims require Institutional Care

An estimated $400 Billions were spent on CVD related health care in 2005, and about $242 Billions were spent in healthcare cost, and $152 Billion in lost productivity Medicare spends about $26 Billion in CVD related Hospitalization cost each year 90% of Middle Aged Americans will develop High Blood Pressure in their life time, and 70% who have it now do not have it controlled. Without adequate measures to prevent Strokes or Brain Attacks will result in a sharp rise in American death rate from Stroke, and a steep rise in "survivors with dependency of one kind or another".

When blood supply in a part of brain is interrupted by blockage of blood vessel or a rupture of blood vessel, thereby allowing the blood to flow in to the brain tissue and resulting in the injury or complete destruction of brain neurons in an area of brain then it is called an incidence of "stroke". If blood supply to the brain is disrupted, brain cells can die or get damaged; it will be identified as "stroke". Stroke is a brain injury caused by death or damage of brain cells and/or neurons. Neurons are responsible for sending messages to all parts of the body, and therefore control just about every function of the body.

Stroke used to be known as ***"Apoplexy"*** which is a Greek word meaning strike down, which is quite literal and appropriate for the incidence of stroke. Stroke is also known as "Cerebral-vascular Accident". Stroke is Brain Attack which occurs in the brain just like Heart Attack which occurs in the heart.

When stroke happens to occur in the left side of the brain, then the right side of the body is effect by paralysis, numbness, inability to function properly, complete disability in some physical functions restrictive movement, insensitivity in some areas, etc. speech, spoken and written language understanding difficulties, etc., etc.

When stroke happens to be in the right side of the brain then the left side of the body is adversely affected, vision is blurred and out of focus, perception and dimensions become unreal, etc. Overall, language, communications abilities, memory, paralysis, etc. are the outcomes of a stroke incidence. Even personality can be altered by a stroke.

Medical community has classified strokes which happen to be of various types. New names would emerge as medical researchers discover new types in the future. Some of these types of strokes have been briefly introduced here.

ISCHEMIC STROKE

It is a common knowledge that blood coagulation is beneficial especially when we are bleeding from a wound. Blood clots are formed with coagulated blood on the damaged site to stop, or at least to slowdown the bleeding, and thereby creating a condition for the wound to heal. On the other hand, blood clots formed from fatty substances, cholesterol, and other elements can block arteries and cut off the flow of blood, which leads to stroke conditions that can be fatal. There are Transient Ischemic Attacks (TIA) which are stroke like attacks resulting from partial blockage of blood vessel in the brain often just for a second or two, resulting in a tremor like, or a blackout like experience just for a second or a fraction of it. This could be called the first warning sign of an oncoming Brain Attack or Stroke in the future. However, if the tremor or blackout lasts longer, an Ischemic stroke occurs causing some damage. An Ischemic Stroke can occur in two ways:

EMBOLIC STROKE

When a blood clot originating from somewhere in the body (quite often from the heart), and then travels through to the brain, and enters into a small blood vessel (tube) and blocks it, embolic stroke occurs, resulting in

20% mortality within 30 days
60% survive the first year, and 50% in 5 year period
60%-70% of survivors suffer some disability
immediately after the stroke
40% in 6 months, and 30% in one year

THROMBOTIC STROKE

When a blood clot forms within the blood vessel locally in the brain, thereby blocking it; this occurrence is called Thrombotic Stroke. This type of blood clot is different from coagulated blood, and is caused by built up of fatty deposits, other substances, and cholesterol. They cause multiple levels of tiny and multiple injuries to the blood vessel walls. The incidence of these injuries gets repeated regularly. Our bodies react to these injuries and tend to repair them. When we are bleeding from a wound our bodies respond by forming blood clots on the wound site to stop bleeding, similarly our bodies form blood clots to repair these injuries, or bleeding inside these injured blood vessels. There are two types of Thrombosis that can cause Stroke: Large Vessel Thrombosis, and Small Vessel Disease.

**LARGE VESSEL THROMBOSIS*

It occurs in the large arteries, and is the best understood one. Most of the time, it is caused by sustained and long term ***Atherosclerosis*** (deposit of plaque is formed by fatty substances on the inner lining of the arterial wall) which promotes rapid blood clot formation by the body. Large Vessel Thrombosis does not show immediate symptoms of injuries to the walls and therefore remain unnoticed for some time during which body continuously forms clots on the damaged site to conduct repairs. Over time one or more pieces of plaque break loose and end up blocking blood vessels in the brain, thereby causing stroke (brain attack). Thrombotic Stroke patients are most likely to have the disease of coronary artery, and heart attack is a common cause of death in patients who have suffered this kind of brain attack or stroke.

**SMALL VESSEL DISEASE*

Small Vessel Disease, also known as ***Lacunars Infarction***, occurs when blood flow is blocked to very small arteries. It is closely linked to hypertension which is caused by high blood pressure, not much is known about this disease

HEMORRHAGIC STROKE

Breakage or blow out of a blood vessel in the brain is Hemorrhagic Stroke, High blood pressure and Cerebral Aneurysm. ***Aneurysm*** is a thin or weak spot on a blood vessel. These weak spots are present at birth, and do not pose any detectable problems until they break. There are two types of Hemorrhagic Strokes.

SUB-ARACHNOID HEMORRHAGE (SAH)

An Aneurism bursts in a large artery on the thin and delicate membrane, or around it that surrounds the brain. As a result of this burst, blood oozes out and spills in to the area around the brain. There is a fluid that surrounds and protects the brain. The spilled blood gets mixed with this protective liquid and contaminates it.

SYMPTOMS OF SUB ARACHNOID HEMORRHAGE (SAH)

*Very severe headache, kind of worst headache.
*Intolerance to light and brightness.
*Stiff neck area.
*Feeling of vomiting and nausea.
*Loss of consciousness.
*Partial loss of vision, speech, understanding, reading and writing etc.
*Partial memory loss.

*Vision impairment.
*Balance, confusion, dizziness, helplessness, feeling of insecurity.
*Sub Arachnoids Hemorrhage has 40% mortality within 30 days of experiencing stroke, 50% of the survivors have disability.

INTRA-CEREBRAL HEMORRHAGE (ICH)

Intra-Cerebral Hemorrhage is when bleeding occurs within a blood vessel in the brain itself. High blood pressure and hypertension are the primary causes of this brain attack, or stroke. It is a major type of stroke.

SYMPTOMS OF INTRA-CEREBRAL HEMORRHAGE (ICH)

Symptoms may vary depending upon the specific location and the amount of bleeding in the brain. However, major symptoms are:

*Excruciating and severe headache like not having experienced before.
*Sudden weakness felt in the legs, joints, arms, face.
*Feeling of nausea, vomiting.
*Partial or total loss of consciousness.
*Balance and coordination.
*Walking difficulties, dizziness.
*Partial memory loss.
*Inability to speak, see, read, keep balance, walk, coordinate, etc.

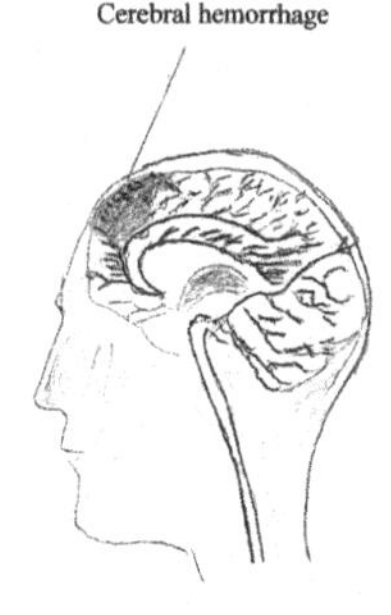

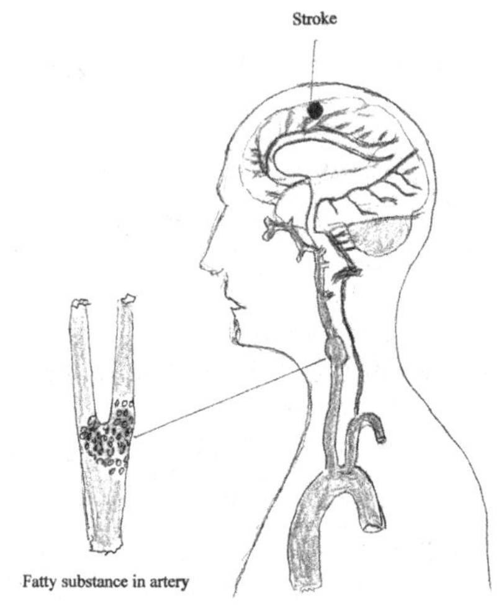

ESSENTIALS FOR THE BRAIN

Regular and smooth flow of blood supply to the brain is crucial to its function. Blood rich in oxygen and other nutrients to feed the brain 24 hours a day via sophisticated system of blood carrying vessels is absolutely essential for the brain to function and stay alive. Brain is 2% of an adult's body weight.
It receives about

20% of body's oxygen
15% of heart's output of fresh blood
100% of liver's output of glucose or blood sugar

Brain has no storage facility, and therefore cannot store any of the above essentials. Ironically, the brain cannot function without these essential elements.

BLOOD CLOT FORMATION

In normal arteries, oxygen rich blood flows smoothly. The arteries remain flexible, and therefore are normal. Cholesterol and plaque accumulate over time in our arteries, and get stuck or lodged to the inner walls of our arteries. The arteries become narrow and this causes the blood flow to get restricted. This causes blood to spurt (somewhat similar to capillary action in the air-conditioning system where the condensed gas passes through a very thin tube (capillary) thereby increasing its pressure therein). Blood flow with some pressure behind it continuously hits the walls of the clogged arteries, which causes rupture. Clogged arteries are when plaque is formed on the inside of the arteries. Spurting of blood with high pressure behind it dislodges some of the plaque and debris is formed. These broken plaque particles clump together with ***platelets***, and other substance in the blood, a blood clot is formed. (Platelets are very tiny elements (cells) of blood, without nuclei, formed in the bone marrow, that initiate blood coagulation through a complicated process).

Although researchers and the medical community consider blood coagulation and blood clotting as one and the same thing, I think they are two different things with some similarities. Coagulation of blood is a natural process of protecting the human body from bleeding to death, that is, through stopping the blood from flowing out of the body from a cut in the skin by thickening or congealing the blood with platelets. Thickened blood with platelets patches the opening of the cut thereby blocking the blood from flowing out of the body. However, the coagulated blood, under extreme dehydrated condition, can become large and block tiny blood vessel in the brain causing a stroke. The blood clots that cause hemorrhages, strokes, and heart attacks are much more than soft blood clots; they are a combination of plaque debris, platelets, and other substance. The blood with platelets, plaque debris and other substance formed in to a blood clot can prove to be deadly. A blood clot in the heart causes a heart attack, and a blood clot in the brain is called a stroke or a brain attack. A blood clot formed with platelets, plaque debris, and other substances in the leg is equally deadly, and is called deep vein thrombosis.

RISK FACTORS

INABILITY TO RECOGNIZE AN ONCOMING STROKE

More than 75% Americans do not know the Symptoms of a Stroke; only 17% of the people know the Symptoms of Stroke to call 911. Knowing about and recognizing the symptoms of an oncoming stroke are crucial to avoiding disability or death from a stroke.

***DEHYDRATION*:**

Dehydration leads to the conditions that cause stroke. Lack of water in the body and therefore in the blood makes the blood thick, and makes it difficult to flow freely. Thickened blood creates a big lump which cannot pass through the tiny blood vessels of the brain, resulting in a stroke. Dehydrated people in dry terrains with the hot sun above can experience a sudden stroke.

HIGH CHOLESTEROL:

Cholesterol is a soft and waxy substance found among the Lipids (fats) in the blood stream and all body cells. It is an important part of a healthy body. Our bodies use Cholesterol to form membranes of all cells, and also some of the hormones, beside other functions

Our bodies have assigned special carriers to transport Cholesterol to and from the body cells. Strangely, Cholesterol and other fats cannot be dissolved in the blood, and therefore either they travel in the blood stream or get stuck and lodged in the walls of arteries. Mainly, there are two kinds of Lipoproteins:

Low Density Lipoproteins (LDL), and
High Density Lipoproteins (HDL)

LDL is the major Cholesterol Carrier in the blood. If too much LDL Cholesterol circulates in the blood, it can slowly build up in the walls of arteries feeding the heart and the brain. LDL in large quantities in the blood stream can join other substances in the blood stream, thereby forming ***plaque*** which is a thick and hard deposit in the walls of arteries. Plaque makes the arteries narrower, and can block arteries. This condition is called ***Atherosclerosis***. A clot that is formed near the plaque is called ***Thrombosis***, which can cause a ***heart attack*** by causing blockage to the heart, or a ***stroke*** by causing blockage of blood flow to the brain. LDL is the Bad Cholesterol, and should be less than 80mg/dl (preferable). Lower level of LDL Cholesterol is better, and reflects a lower risk of Stroke.

HDL carries about one third of the Blood Cholesterol in our bodies. Medical experts think that HDL tends to carry Cholesterol away from the arteries, and bring back to the liver where it is passed through the body. While, other Medical experts believe that HDL removes excess Cholesterol from the plaque and slows down their growth. HDL seems to protect our bodies from Stroke and Heart Attack. HDL is the good Cholesterol. High HDL level is good for our bodies. We enter a **high risk zone** when our HDL is

Less than 50mg/dl for Women

Less than 40mg/dl for men

and therefore low HDL level in our body is definitely a High Risk factor for us.

LP (a)-Cholesterol is a variation of plasma LDL. High level of LP (a) Cholesterol is an important Risk Factor for developing ***Atherosclerosis* prematurely. Lesions in the walls of arteries contain substances that may interact with LP (a) which stimulate building up of fatty deposits. Above 80mg/dl of LDL will take women to the Risk Zone.

Our body produces 1000 mgs of Cholesterol each and every day. We do not need additional cholesterol at all, but we cannot avoid it under the current lifestyle. It is recommended that we should take less than 300 mgs per day from the food source for healthy individuals, and less than 200 mgs per day from the food source for Stroke and Heart patients. Smoke lowers the HDL (good cholesterol) levels, and it increases the tendency for the blood to clot. Alcohol increases the HDL (good cholesterol) levels in the body, but should be consumed in moderation only due to its adverse affect on the liver.

All animal products have cholesterol. Some of them are: eggs, beef, chicken, pork, shrimp, etc., and the foods that have high saturated fats or Trans fatty acids are: grilled cheese sandwiches, margarine, chicken salad, etc. Cholesterol from foods enters your digestive track, and then it reaches your liver, and from there it can easily circulate throughout the body via the bloodstream.

Also, our body produces cholesterol naturally, and our family history, Genes, play a significant role in this process. Most of the cholesterol in the blood stream comes from our own body, which is essential for the maintenance of our physical system. When our intakes of foods that are high in cholesterol are added to the cholesterol which our body has naturally produced, the result is high cholesterol. Muscle weakness or any other weakness that cannot be explained must be attended to immediately, as this could be the result of High Cholesterol levels and possibly some blockage in the flow of blood.

PLAQUE

Plaque is a combination of cholesterol, other fatty substances, calcium, and blood elements, and this combination of components stick together to the artery wall lining. Over a period of time, a hard shell forms called plaque. Plaques have various sizes and shapes. There are hard and somewhat softer Plaques. The unstable and softer Plaques can rupture or burst open, thereby causing blood clotting inside the artery. If a blood clot ends up blocking the artery completely, it can stop the flow of blood completely resulting in stroke or heart attack.

The exact causes of ***Atherosclerosis*** are not completely clear and defined. It could be a combination of causes like: too much cholesterol in the blood, damage to the arterial wall, inflammation, etc that play important role in plaque build up. Researches are studying how plaque actually develops and changes over time, how the arteries become damaged, and why Plaque can burst and break open giving way to blood clot formation. Although the exact causes are not definable, but there are some indicators which are directly related to it.

LIFESTYLE

-High blood cholesterol through eating fatty foods
-Over weight and obesity gained through uncontrolled eating and drinking.
-Maintaining lethargic lifestyle with no exercise.
-High blood pressure
-Eating and sleeping disorders

HYPERTENSION

Hypertension is often described as the Silent Killer. It is caused by:

-Anxiety caused by various life circumstances
-When the pressure in the Arteries is building up, slowly or rapidly
-Heart is working harder than normal

-Blood vessels are constricted and holding back the flow of blood due to high stress levels and continuous anxiety
-Extra wear and tear of blood vessels, and causing certain areas to
weaken, which become vulnerable points for stroke to occur
-High Blood Pressure.

AGE FACTOR

-Arteries become fragile with age
-Arteries become less elastic, less flexible, and become hardened
-Lack of elasticity and flexibility in the hardened Arteries drives them to get clogged
-Decrease in body liquid as we age

DIABETES

-Diabetics are three times more likely to have a stroke
-They are twice more likely to have hypertension
-42% Stroke Patients also have diabetes
-Diabetics are more prone to high cholesterol, and obesity.

FAMILY HISTORY

We all know now that genes play the most important role in our lives. Genes create a physical destiny in our lives, and it seems that we are captive to this design of nature. If we carry a family history of cardio vascular disease, (CVD), or high blood pressure (HBP) then the probability is very high of experiencing physical damage from these diseases. By proper precautions, healthy lifestyle and medication, we can delay such occurrences for several years at least, if not for decades.

TOBACCO

Tobacco smoking lowers the HDL (good cholesterol) levels in the body, increases the tendency for the blood to clot. Nicotine and carbon monoxide reduces the oxygen in blood, also they damage the walls of blood vessels, thereby creating a condition for clots to form. Birth control pills and tobacco smoking increase the chances of having a stroke. Smoking tobacco provides the smoker a supply of about 4,000 compounds of chemicals, and is the leading cause of stroke/heart disease. It damages the coronary arteries, harms the aorta, and causes sudden stroke/heart attack.

Smoking tobacco provides adequate supply of nicotine, nitrosamine, tar, pesticides, carbon monoxide, volatile organic compounds, (benzene), cadmium (metal), radio active polonium (metal), carbonyl compounds, polycyclic aromatic hydro carbons, etc, a total of about 400 carbons in tobacco smoking that are lethal to humans.

RECOMMENDATIONS

*Healthy lifestyle with regular exercise and adequate diet.
*Avoid dehydration by drinking lots of water daily.
*Eliminating abuse of alcohol and food.
*Avoiding tobacco smoking and smoke environment.
*Controlling and regulating stress, anger, diet, sleep, and blood pressure.

*Avoiding confrontations of all kinds.
*Regular and scheduled meditation.
*Social activity participation
*Developing and maintaining helpful and kind disposition toward others.

*To heal from a stroke condition, or to avoid having one, the most prominent areas to consider will be to cut down all the deep fried foods in your diet, which can be avoided. It is difficult to cut down all the fatty foods that we have been accustomed to eating all our lives, however, occasional consumption of favorite foods, in small portions only, prepared with caution, may be consumed.

*Saturated fat intake should be minimized. Butter, margarine, whole milk, meat, poultry with skin, etc. are loaded with saturated fats and cholesterols and increased consumption of these foods can cause severe health problems. Minimize or eliminate saturated fats from your diet. Develop a taste for vegetarian foods and a habit of using olive oil in you cooking.

*Eliminate foods containing Trans Fatty acids (AA) which are plentiful in vegetable shortening and margarine and in the products made with partially hydrogenated oils. Develop taste for foods that contain Omega-3 fatty acids, and increase their consumption frequency. Omega-3 fatty acids are sufficiently found in fish oil, flax seed oil, and flaxseed meal. Just watch the adequate ratio of omega-6 and omega-3 fatty acids when consuming fish. Only certain fish are good.

*For clean arteries and adequate blood circulation, certain practices can be of immense help to your maintaining a healthy body. If onions, garlic, ginger, cayenne peppers, paprika, lime, vinegar, whole grains, beans, lentils, olive oil, fat free milk, tofu, a variety of vegetables and fruits covering all ranges of color, oat bran and wheat bran, green or processed tea, and maintaining a healthy life style under non toxic environment are not a part of your current daily life then make every effort to incorporate them in anything and everything you eat and do.

*Eat wheat bran which contains non-soluble fiber that cleans the intestinal walls. Eat Oat bran which contains water soluble fiber which removes the cholesterol from the blood, which in turn, lowers the blood pressure. This is one good way to avoid having a stroke or a heart attack.

*People feel proud realizing that they are on the top of food chain on this planet. Just avoid being on top of the food chain. Eat foods that are on the lower chain of life. Foods that are on higher chain of life not only contain high quantities of total fat, and saturated fats, but also contain various chemicals, herbicides, pesticides, heavy metals, and other toxins which happen to be extremely toxic and dangerous to humans. If possible, avoid animal products completely, or consume them marginally.

*Are we pre-ordained for our experiences? Not really. If there was no food, then humans would be eating vegetation to survive, and there was no medical help then humans will do whatever it takes to stay alive and healthy. Of course, not too many would survive without medical help if a major disease came upon us. But most of us would try our best to survive, because we all have been genetically endowed with the ***instinct to survive***. Most certainly, we do not have to abandon this instinct to survive under modern conditions where a significant amount of medical help is available and can be sought.

This is the very instinct that helps most people to survive under unbearable and adverse conditions. Why can't we use this natural gift of survival under modern conditions when abundant food and medical help are available? In spite of this affluence, people still die. In fact, medical help cannot guarantee life, longevity, or good health to any one on this planet, whether it happens to be a human or any other species of animal kingdom. We should never succumb to the thought that if medical help did not arrive, or is not available for one reason or another, it is the end of the world. Without our individual desire and will to survive, even the best medical help cannot help us. It is within us that instigate the survival process, and it has never existed outside of our mind. Please do remember this because this is the only thing that will help you survive a Stroke, or any other serious health condition, no matter how sophisticated medical help you may receive during a very trying period of Stroke. Medical community and research institutes are becoming aware of the fact that medicines help to boost the immune system of the body, and once the immune system is good and running the body cures the health problem itself. Medicines help to boost the immune system, but do not cure the ailment. Here, the ***patients' will to get better***, and active participation become of prime importance.

*Exercise by walking daily as much as you can, and/or participating in some light exercise routine which you can easily maintain on a regular basis, hopefully throughout your life should be adopted.

*Learning to recognize the symptoms of an oncoming stroke and to manage it will save your life, and possibly spare you from being hauled away in an ambulance and examined and treated by an inexperienced, unknown doctor, or by unsympathetic medical staff members, or from an unnecessary surgical procedure, or from lifelong disability.

Knowledge of Stroke symptoms could bring you closer to avoiding it; however, ignorance could bring you closer to death or disability.

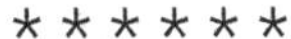

HEART DISEASE

Heart disease kills as many women as men, if not more. Most women are not aware of their risk of suffering from heart disease. Each year, cardiovascular disease (heart disease and stroke) kills about ten times more women than breast cancer. As the stress levels of working women increase, which is inevitable due to their increasingly responsible position in the working world in the future, the incidence of heart disease and other cardiovascular diseases will increase. Current estimates indicate that more than 230,000 women die of heart disease each year in America, and a huge number end up with disability

Heart is a hollow muscle about the size of your fist. It's like a pumping machine which is fitted with all the essential pipes to pump blood. Heart pumps about 5 quarts of blood through your body each and every minute, by means of regular and forceful contraction and expansion of its 4 chambers. Each thump of the heart is participated by the upper chamber, called ***atria***, and the lower chamber, called the ***ventricles***, means 2 beats. The heart beats about 70 beats a minute, or more than two and half billion beats in a lifetime of 70 years. The heart is divided in to left and right by a solid muscular wall, called the ***septum*** which prevents the blood in two sides from mixing.

The right side of the heart receives the used blood from the veins and pumps it to the lungs for the filtering and recycling process. The lungs take away the carbon dioxide from the blood and provide oxygen to the blood through exhaling and inhaling of air. The left side of heart receives fresh blood with oxygen from the lungs and pumps it throughout the body through blood vessels. The heart requires a continuous flow of nutrients and oxygen to maintain its own health and survival. If heart is deprived of nutrients, oxygen, or an infection causes it to weaken, a variety of heart related health problems occur.

Heart disease is the number one threat to women. About 230,000 women die of heart disease each year in the United States, and about 48% die before reaching the hospital. Almost half of the fatalities were due to the delay in recognizing the symptoms of an oncoming heart disease related occurrence. Here are some of the prominent heart disease related health conditions for you to get familiarize with:

STABLE ANGINA

When too much stress is exerted on the body too suddenly, in a short span of time, an angina attack may occur. Sudden strenuous exercise or an activity demands a lot of blood to be pumped out of the heart causing it an excessive stress which can damage the heart or bring about a heart attack. During a snowstorm, stepping out of the house and feverishly shoveling snow to clear the driveway, or jogging in the spring after passing the winter inactively, etc may bring about a '***chest pain***' or '***chest discomfort***' which is caused by over exerted heart. Each winter and springtime, many people are taken to the hospitals, some don't return.

UNSTABLE ANGINA

Unstable angina is term for a severe pain in the chest which is caused by insufficient supply of blood to the heart. Reduced supply of blood to the heart is caused by narrowing of arteries to the heart. Its occurrence is very painful, and the patient feels dizzy, and sweaty.

CONGENITAL HEART DISEASE

*Congenital heart disease relates to abnormal heart by birth. ***Congenital heart blockage*** occurs when there is interference in the electrical nerve impulses which regulate the rhythmic pumping activity of the heart muscle. When the two upper chambers of the heart beat normally, but the two lower chambers lag behind and are out of sync, or beat abnormally.

*There may be ***septal defects*** which refer to the holes in the wall dividing the left and right sides of the heart chamber.

*Another heart defect is **pulmonary stenosis** which refers to a condition in which one of the 4 heart valves—pulmonary valve—is so narrow that blood flow to the lungs is restricted.

*Yet, another condition is ***patent ductus arteriosus,*** which allows some freshly oxygenated blood that is headed for the body leaks back in to the pulmonary artery which places added strain to the heart. All these conditions are treatable and non-life threatening.

CORONARY HEART DISEASE

Coronary heart disease is best described when the coronary arteries become narrow due to the formation of plaque within the arterial walls, and cause stoppage or reduce the flow of blood to the heart muscle which, in most cases, results in heart attack. There are several causes which affect the coronary arteries and the heart muscle. Reduced blood flow is caused by ***arteriosclerosis*** which is referred to the overall arterial health condition. Arteries have several layers of walls within. Healthy arteries are elastic, but over time and with unhealthy habits, the elasticity of these walls gets reduced. The arteries lose elasticity and become hard hence the common term hardening of arteries is often applied for arteriosclerosis. ***Atherosclerosis*** is one of several kinds of arteriosclerosis. It's a degenerative change in the arterial walls of arteries, primarily the larger ones: aorta, coronary, and cerebral vessels, which causes the narrowing of the arteries. Narrowing of arteries is caused by plaque formation on the inner walls of the blood vessels.

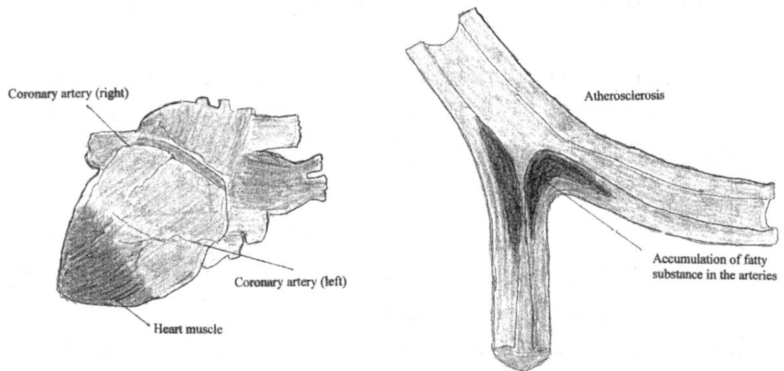

HEART ATTACK

Heart attack is term given to the condition when the coronary artery is blocked with a blood clot and the flow of blood is stopped to the heart. Most of the time, it results in a quick death. However, if the clot is bit smaller, which allows some blood to pass through to the heart a severe damage to the heart muscle occurs and diminishes its ability to function properly. The damage may occur elsewhere as well due to disruption of blood supply. If the supply of blood is blocked or restricted, the cells of heart muscle die, which weakens it. When heart muscle weakens due to lack of sufficient nutrients and oxygen, invariably it gets damaged and its performance becomes less than adequate. Heart attack is also known as ***coronary thrombosis*** which literally means the blockage of coronary artery by a blood clot.

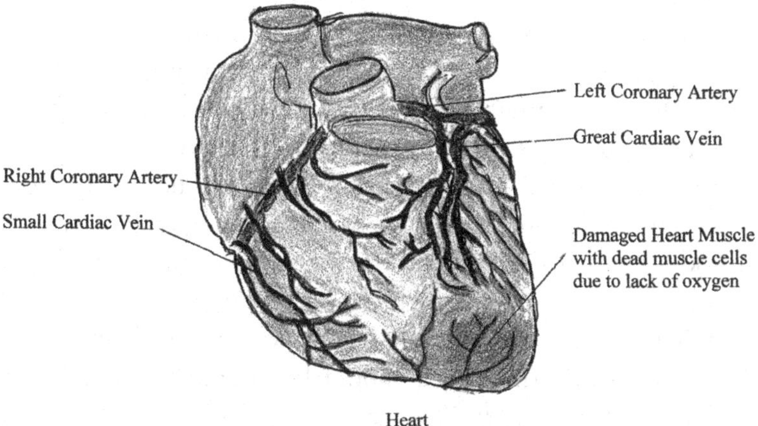

Heart

HEART FAILURE

Heart failure occurs when the heart muscles fail to pump as much blood as it needs to. Your body will respond to this emergency of short supply automatically and take protective measures. The body increases the heart rate, the size of the heart is increased, and it conserves the salt and water to increase the supply of blood in the blood stream. These are emergency measures taken by the body, but it lasts for a very short time only.

CARDIOMYOPATHY

Cardiomyopathy is any disease of the heart muscle, which deteriorates and weakens the heart muscle. Weakened heart muscle puts patients at risk of sudden death, or loss of consciousness.

ARRHYTHMIA

Arrhythmia is a condition which is referred to the heart beat's timing and accuracy. When the heart beat is too slow, or too fast, or it skips a beat occasionally is called arrhythmia. (For example, heart beating at 60 beats per minute is too slow, and 100 beats per minute is too fast). When the heart beat is faster than normal it is called ***tachycardia***, and when it is slower than normal it is called ***bradycardia***. It is normally not a serious condition, unless the heart beat is way too fast or way too slow. There are many causes for the heart beat to fluctuate and lose its rhythm, which include coronary heart disease, abnormal hormonal balance, blood chemistry imbalance, and certain medications. You should be alarmed if your heart starts beating rapidly and you experience a pounding and thumping with palpitation.

SYMPTOMS

Since women were never considered as candidates for heart disease, very little if any research materials were developed on their health condition. Until recently, heart disease was a man's disease. Women have been having a hard time being heard of their problems by the medical community who have been schooled and trained to think that symptoms of men are standards that should apply to women as well. There are some differences in the symptoms and therefore the treatment must be somewhat different too.

*Women experience palpitation during resting or active period- gradually or suddenly.
*Women get sensation of dizziness and approaching unconsciousness.
*Women feel chest pains, shortness of breath, over whelming fatigue, chills, pain in both arms, shoulders and back, sudden dizziness or loss of consciousness, a sense of impending doom, and squeezing chest pain.

WOMEN AT HIGH RISK

*Women with history of stroke, heart disease, vascular disease in legs, abdominal aorta, aneurysm, and chronic kidney disease have more than 20% chance of experiencing an occurrence of stroke, heart attack, or death within 10 years, according *American Heart Association*.
*Women with calcium in the coronary arteries, metabolic syndrome, multiple heart risk factors, and family history of early heart disease have between 10% to 20% chance of experiencing an occurrence of stroke, heart attack, or death within 10 years after diagnosis, according to *American Heart Association*.

*Women with low levels of HDL (high density lipoprotein) are at high risk of heart disease and related death.
*Post menopausal women under hormone replacement therapy have high risk of heart attack and death from coronary artery disease.
*Women heart attack patients going to the hospital have twice the death rate that of men. *Women experience more complications during and after the heart attack.
*Menopausal women with heart attack have twice the death rate than men.

MENOPAUSAL WOMEN & RISK FACTORS

As women approach menopause, the production of estrogen (female hormone) is somewhat reduced. Ovaries start producing lesser quantities of estrogen, which cause changes in the menstrual cycles beside some other physical changes. The most common symptoms of menopause are:

*night sweating
*dryness in vagina
*hot flashes
*emotional changes

Menopause occurs naturally between the ages 45 to 55. If ovaries have been removed then loss of estrogen will occur. Loss of estrogen can also occur if a woman experiences an early menopause.

*Loss of natural estrogen or less natural estrogen as women age contributes to higher risk of heart disease.
*After the menopause, there is remarkable change in the walls of blood vessels, and plaque starts building up. Plaque formation is the start of blood clot formation.
*Menopause affects the HDL and LDL levels in the bloodstream. After menopause, the HDL decreases and LDL increases in the blood which is a warning call for all women.
*Increased levels of fibrinogen (blood clotting substance in the blood) to clot more than before, thereby elevating the risk of stroke and heart attack.

**Menopausal women should stop smoking, because
tobacco smoking decreases the supply of oxygen to the heart
it increases the blood pressure
it increases blood clotting
it damages cells in the coronary arteries, and other blood vessels.

Department of Health & Human Services reports that 42% of women who suffered from heart attack die within 1 year, as compared to 24% of men. Additionally, women may not be diagnosed or treated as aggressively as men.

RECOMMENDATIONS

*Give up smoking tobacco, and the smoke environment.
*Maintain healthy weight.
*Perform regular exercise.
*Eat heart healthy diet which includes fruits, vegetables, nuts, legumes, lentils, grains, tea, some chocolate, and some red wine.
*Drink a lot of water, that is, more than 8 glasses each day.
*Maintain waistline of less than 35 inches, and BMI (bone mass index) of 18.5 to 24.9.

*Get checked regularly, including for depression.
*Take omega-3 supplement.
*Maintain blood pressure at 120/80 mm Hg.
*Control blood sugar by eliminating sweets and commercial sugars.
*Maintain LDL cholesterol at 80mg/dl (preferably) and HDL at higher than 50 mg/dl.
*Maintain triglycerides at less than 150 mg/dl.
*Maintain cholesterol levels less than 180.
*Consult your doctor regularly.
*Maintain a happy social life.
*Make efforts to remove stress from your life.

*You should prepare yourself for heart attack: calling 911 procedures, selection of right hospital, ambulance response time, HDL/LDL levels, and list of current medications, current allergies, and the results of screening should be kept

handy, as recommended by Dr. Bob Arnold in his book *(Seven steps to stop heart attack)*
*Consume as many leafy vegetables and fruits as you can each and every day, because they contain thousands of antioxidants that protect and enhance body's immune system.

*Sleep at least for 7 hours each day. Inadequate or lack of sleep is a stress signal to the body which responds by releasing stress hormones such as ***cortisol*** and ***norepinephrine***, which constrict the arteries and increase bloodstream sugar levels, causing inflammation.
*Attend to the wellbeing and optimal functioning of other organs of your body. The health of your heart is directly related to the health of other organs in your body. Body organs work in harmony, and they respond to each other in every sense of the word. This goes for organ transplant as well. Transplant success depends upon the health condition of all other organs in the patient's body. Newly transplanted organ can be rejected by the body if other organs are not healthy.

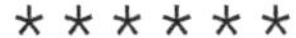

LIVER DISEASES

Liver is among the largest organs, and performs some of the most vital functions of the body. Most of it is located in the upper right of the abdomen, and a portion extends up to the middle left of the body.

LIVER FUNCTIONS

*Liver metabolizes protein, fats, minerals, and carbohydrates.
*Filters blood.
*Makes an important protein "***albumin***" which regulates fluid transport in the blood and the kidneys. (Albumin is sulfur containing soluble protein which coagulates when heated
*Makes bile which helps the digestion of fats, and excretes certain fatty substances.

*Converts glucose to glycogen, and stores it as a source of energy.
*Stores iron, copper, Vitamins A, D, and several of B family.
*Removes or processes toxins that enter the body through food intake, breathing, and the environment we live and work in.
*Makes the essential elements necessary for blood clotting.

*Destroys the old red blood cells and converts hemoglobin molecules in to ***Bilirubin.***

CAUSES & RISK FACTORS

Bacterial invasion, viral infection, physical or chemical change in the body, and malnutrition can impair the functioning of the liver. The most common cause of liver damage is malnutrition, especially through alcoholism. Liver diseases can cause ***liver failure***, ***cirrhosis***, and illness in other parts of the body, beside ***kidney failure***, ***low blood count***, ***gastro-intestinal bleeding***, ***encephalopathy*** (deterioration of the brain function which leads to coma), ***peptic ulcers*** (which erode ***stomach lining), esophageal varices (bleeding from esophagus), liver cancer***, etc. Liver diseases are highly contagious and pose threats to others through foods, water, and sexual contacts.

Each year, more than 400,000 new cases are reported, and the patients who survive from disability or death are the ones who contacted the medical community in time, that is, during earlier stages.

SYMPTOMS OF LIVER DISEASE

*Yellowing of skin.
*Dark urine.
*Weight loss or weight gain.
*Nausea, vomiting, diarrhea.
*Loss of appetite.
*Light colored stools.
*Pain in the upper right part of the stomach.
*General itching.
*Some feeling of illness.
*Varicose veins,

*Fatigue, hypoglycemia (low sugar),
*Muscle aches and pains,
*Low grade fever,
*Depression.

Some of the well known liver diseases are briefly described below:

JAUNDICE

Jaundice is the most common source of problems with the liver. It is caused by the excessive amounts of bile pigment (***bilirubin***) in the blood stream and all the body tissues of the body. This causes yellowing of the skin, which is called Jaundice. Inflammation is caused by excessive sugars, toxins, infections, and injuries in the liver. Once inflammation occurs in the liver, the small bile duct through which ***bilirubin*** is excreted out gets blocked. ***Bilirubin***, a natural bi-product of the red blood cells in the liver, is a concoction of bile and other digestive juices. If the outflow of the bile is restricted and blocked; ***bilirubin*** cannot flow out to the small intestines from where it would have traveled to the anus to be expelled out of the body. Instead, ***bilirubin*** remains in the liver and gets absorbed in to the blood stream, creating an excessive supply of bile pigments.

Jaundice in children is generally not very serious; however, in adults it spells various serious health problems.

HEPATITIS

In general, it is inflammation of the liver caused by viral infection commonly known as hepatitis A, B, C, and D. Another type of hepatitis is caused by toxicity from the environment, alcohol abuse, use of drugs, etc. Its symptoms resemble that of flu, and therefore it is often misdiagnosed. It is estimated that at least 500,000 people in the USA have this disease. It is dangerous because it interferes with many functions of the liver. Although most patients recover from this disease, however, it can lead to ***cirrhosis***, and possibly death.

Hepatitis A is contracted through food, water, or fecal contamination. It is the least dangerous type. Improper handling of food, unhygienic conditions, polluted water, etc. cause this virus.

Hepatitis B is the most widespread disease. More than 300,000 people get infected each year in the USA Hepatitis B can spread through mother to child, within the family, through sexual contact, sharing needles, intravenous drug use, etc. Only 1% to 2% of the patients die of this disease, however, many develop ***cirrhosis***.

Hepatitis C spreads through contact with blood or through contaminated needles. 30% of chronic patients develop cirrhosis.

Hepatitis D infects only patients with Hepatitis B. It can be transmitted from mother to child, and also through sexual contact. It involves two forms of disease working at once and, therefore, it is very dangerous.

Hepatitis E occurs mainly in Asia, Africa, and Mexico. Only time it is identified in the United States is when someone has brought it from overseas, otherwise it does not exist here. For pregnant women, Hepatitis E is considered to be very dangerous.

Environmental toxicity, alcohol & drug abuse causes

the inflammation of the liver, and does not have any viral infection. Excessive and chronic consumption of prescription and over the counter drugs are also inflammatory and cause liver problems.

CIRRHOSIS

Liver cells die of viral hepatitis, alcoholism, toxic chemicals, prolonged obstruction of bile, genetic deficiencies, etc, and cease to function. Lack of cell activity among dead cells causes them to dry out, and the formation of fibrous tissue results, which is known as cirrhosis. Symptoms appear until the late stages.

SYMPTOMS OF CIRRHOSIS include jaundice, dark urine, dark or bloody stools, swollen legs or feet, fatigue, loss of stamina, abdomen swelling, menstrual disturbances, nausea, sleep disturbances, red palms, etc. Without proper treatment, cirrhosis can cause death.

CHRONIC CIRRHOSIS of the liver creates grounds for parasitic invasion. Cysts of the liver are usually caused by parasitic infestation by ***echinococcus***. Cysts may grow slowly over time and become calcified which is a very serious health condition requiring surgery. Almost all parasitic infestations in the body, such as tuberculosis, leprosy, etc. can affect the liver resulting in swelling or damage to the liver cells.

RECOMMENDATIONS FOR CIRRHOSIS

*Although it is best not to drink alcohol at all, however, the safe limit for women is one or maximum two alcoholic drinks per day depending upon several other factors.
*Maintain a healthy and balanced diet with regularity, and don't skip meals.

*Stay away from industrial chemical environment, because chemicals can get in you and then in your blood stream, which can cause liver damage.

*Take precautions against contracting hepatitis, and if possible get shots for hepatitis before traveling overseas.
*Practice safe sex.
*Avoid eating uncooked shellfish.
*Alcohol and drugs don't go together; therefore never mix them because some drugs can cause reaction which may result in liver damage.

HEMOCHROMATOSIS

When abnormal amounts of iron get deposited on the liver (and other organs) causing it to function improperly, the color of the skin changes to bronze like. This may indicate that the liver has not been able to absorb all the iron, or excrete the excess amount. It's a progressive disease and requires medical attention without delay. One of the treatments to cure ***hemochromatosis*** is blood letting to deplete the iron stored in the body.

WILSON'S DISEASE

Wilson's disease causes the body to retain copper in the body, which otherwise would get excreted. Excessive amounts of copper damages kidneys, brain, and eyes, causes liver disease, liver failure, cirrhosis, and hepatitis.

SYMPTOMS OF WILSON'S DISEASE are tremors of head, arms, legs; difficulty in swallowing, impaired muscle tone, abnormal posture, slurred speech, clumsiness, and loss of motor skills. Some patients may play out improper behavior, and experience neurosis, psychosis, and depression. Medical help must be sought immediately to determine the copper levels in the body. If untreated, the patients may face liver failure, brain damage, or death.

PRIMARY SCLEROSING CHOLANGITIS

Primary sclerosing cholangitis is a chronic and progressive disease of the bile ducts that drain from the liver to the upper portion of the small intestine. Over time, these ducts can get inflamed, scarred, and narrowed, and finally get obstructed. The obstructed or blocked ducts cause a back up in the liver, and causes abdominal pain, jaundice, itching, infection in the bile ducts (cholangitis), and scarring of the liver. This condition eventually develops in to cirrhosis of the liver and liver failure.

PRIMARY BILIARY CIRRHOSIS

Primary biliary cirrhosis refers to the inflammatory destruction of the small bile ducts within the liver. This condition invariably leads to the cirrhosis of the liver. 90% of patients are women. As the area of the scar tissue increases with the progression of this disease, liver loses its functionality. Also, the established cirrhosis prevents the blood from returning to the heart. It is an autoimmune disease of the small bile ducts.

SYMPTOMS OF PRIMARY BILIARY CIRRHOSIS are itching on the skin of arms, legs, and the back, fluid build up in abdomen and ankles. Appearance of yellowish skin color, yellowish eyes, or a full fledged jaundice means that the disease has progressed. Primary biliary cirrhosis can cause dry eyes, dry mouth, arthritis, thyroid condition, gallstones, and bone fractures.

BUDD CHIARI SYNDROME

Budd chiari syndrome is referred to when the blood clots completely or partially block the large veins (***hepatic veins***) that carry blood from the liver.

Some patients have no ***SYMPTOMS***, and some experience jaundice, fatigue, abdominal pain, accumulation of fluids in the abdomen, nausea, and in some cases severe bleeding in the esophagus. Blood flow out of the liver gets restricted due to the blood clots in the large veins, causing it to enlarge. The blood pressure in the portal vein increases because of the back up of blood in the hepatic veins, which can lead to the formation of varicose veins in the esophagus known as ***esophageal varices***. The blood clots may also block the large vein which carries blood from the lower part of the body to the heart. Also, varicose veins near the skin surface of the abdomen may develop. Consequently, severe cirrhosis of the liver occurs. Other causes include excess number of red blood cells, sickle cell disease, inflammatory bowel disease, or an injury.

GILBERT'S SYNDROME

It is a liver disorder, and a genetic one. When the liver fails to process the substance called ***bilirubin***, produced by the breakdown of the red blood cells, the levels of bilirubin rise resulting in a mild jaundice. About 7% of the entire population experiences it. It is not a dangerous health condition but, nevertheless, requires medical attention.

GLYCOGEN STORAGE DISEASE type II

Build up glycogen (principal carbohydrate storage material chiefly in the liver) causes progressive muscle weakness throughout the body affecting heart, skeletal muscles, liver, and nervous system.

LIVER CANCER

Liver filters blood on a continuous basis. It converts nutrients in to chemicals which can be used by the body for its nourishment. It removes chemical waste products and a variety of toxins from the blood, and makes them ready for the excretion. Cancer cells, present in the blood stream, will pass through the liver or colonize there. For some unknown reason, the liver is unable to clean itself.

Most liver cancers originate from elsewhere such as breast, lung, and colon. The primary cancer which starts from within the liver accounts for more than 50% of all cancers in the under-developed and developing countries while, here in the United States the incidence is little when compared to all types of cancers. But women with Hepatitis, a contagious virus, and/or Cirrhosis predispose them for liver cancer.

CAUSES OF LIVER CANCER

The primary causes of liver cancer are linked to hepatitis B and C, cirrhosis, ***hemochromatosis*** (excessive iron in the liver), some cholesterol lowering drugs, some herbicides, ***aflatoxins*** (develop naturally in stored foods), and chemicals like arsenic, vinyl chloride, and athletic performance improvement drugs, etc. ***Aflatoxins,*** a potent carcinogen produced by fungus in the soil, develop naturally in grains, seeds, nuts, rice, etc as they age, especially in humid environment, has been linked to liver cancer by researchers.

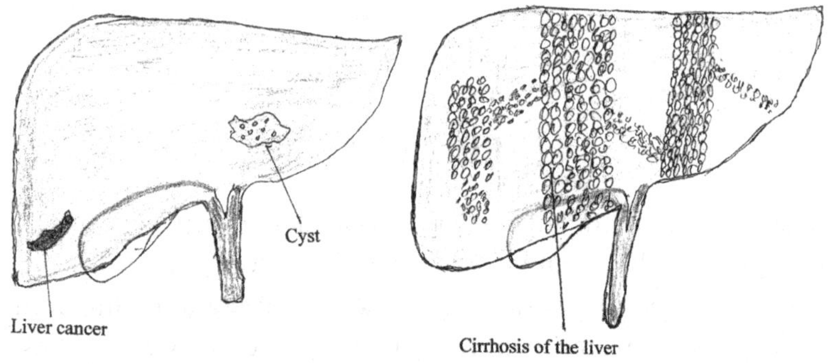

RECOMMENDATIONS

*Drink alcohol only in moderation, and none if you are a patient of liver disease
*If possible, get immunized against hepatitis B
*Let the doctor decide if you need iron supplements, and in what doses.
*Follow guidelines if you work in an environment of cancer causing chemicals
*Talk to your doctor regarding use of athletic performance improvement drugs.

*Check inside of your pantry if some grains, seeds, nuts, etc have been sitting there for years under humid conditions in loosely capped containers. If so, discard them, because ***aflatoxins*** develop naturally in foods stored in damp conditions. All foods should be stored in airtight containers in a cool place.
*Eat yogurt and pickled vegetables every day to maintain beneficial bacteria in the body.
*Drink lots of clean water, that is, more than 8 glasses every day.
*Good hygiene is the primary precaution that all women should take and make it a practice. Frequently washing hands and using only the clean towels to dry, maintaining sanitary

conditions in kitchen, bathroom, and all other areas of the dwelling, and generally keeping the body clean in every possible manner are some of the basic measures every woman should take.

*Taking extreme care while visiting a foreign country, especially regarding eating and drinking, because Americans have lost immunity to a variety of bacteria and viruses to which many people in other countries are immune to.

*A well balanced diet, avoiding alcohol abuse and illegal drugs, and not sharing your personal use articles like combs, scissors, nail-clippers, drinking glass, etc. are some of the additional precautions every woman should take.

*If you have had hepatitis A then, with your physician's advice, getting the immune globulin injection, and fully completing any and every prescription of medicine may prove to be extra protective measure.

*Additionally, try your best to avoid exposure to industrial areas, and environments of fumes, gases, chemicals, herbicides, pesticides, fungicides, etc.

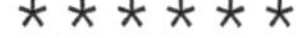

KIDNEY DISEASE

The kidneys are two fist sized organs, located on either side in the back just above the waist line, perform remarkable task of cleaning the blood. Kidneys act like a filtration plant for removing waste and other substances from the blood, thereby maintaining a healthy balance of body chemicals. About 1,700 quarts of blood flow through the kidneys every day, but only one thousands of it is converted in to urine. Kidneys produce the urine, and the urinary passageways dispose it off. The system of filtration and excretion is carried out by more than 1,000,000 ***nephrons*** in each kidney. Nephrons are microscopic urine forming filters which are uniquely shaped and tightly packed in the thick outer part of each kidney.

Under normal conditions, only small sized waste contents filter through the nephrons, and protein and some other substance are left behind. Waste gets through the filtration process and becomes urine, and protein and other substances remain in the bloodstream.

Excessive levels of sugars, starches, and carbohydrates in the bloodstream drive the kidneys to work abnormally long, which makes them tired and weak. Over extended period of time, these unique filters begin to leak, allowing some protein to pass through and appear in the urine, which will establish the condition as 'kidney disease'. This also means that from here on, unless medically attended to, the kidneys will be progressively losing their filtration capabilities, which will lead to the accumulation of waste products inside the bloodstream causing even more dangerous health conditions leading to kidney failure.

Heart disease is the major cause of death for women with kidney disease which is closely linked to hypertension also. Persistent protein in the urine is a definite sign of presence of kidney disease. 26 million Americans have this disease.

CAUSES OF KIDNEY DISEASE

*Diabetes:** all types of diabetic conditions affect the function of kidneys and their malfunction, cause diseases and kidney failure.

Atherosclerosis: it impedes the flow of blood inside the kidneys.

*Inflammation:** it causes abnormality in the function of kidneys, and causes damage to it through over stimulating the body's immune system.

*Blood pressure:** fluctuation in the blood pressure causes disruption and offsets the balance in the kidney function, and depletes the blood supply inside it intermittently.

*Diet:** some researchers believe that excessive amounts of protein and vitamin-D can harm the kidneys.

*Genetics**: inherited genes predispose you to get kidney disease.

****Drugs and toxins**: legal drugs, illegal drugs, and chemicals put an extra burden on the kidneys and cause them to malfunction. Aspirin, analgesics, acetaminophen, etc are some of the drugs become burdensome on kidneys.

****Alcohol and excessive sug**ar can cause overload on the kidneys functionality, and cause them to malfunction.

****Dehydration:** long time without liquids can cause serious damage to the kidneys which can get dehydrated and clogged.

****Athletic injury**: long distance running can break down the muscle tissue, which releases a chemical called ***myoglobin*** (hemoglobin of muscles, but weighing less and carrying more oxygen and less carbon monoxide than hemoglobin). It can damage the kidneys, leading them to failure.

KIDNEY STONES

Urine is a saturated solution of many substances including minerals. Stones are formed from dissolved substances. Some of them condense on a speck of mucus and grow larger. There is no precise pattern as to why stones are formed in one woman and not the other, why women in one part of the United States are more susceptible to having kidney stones and not other.

If some stones are lodged inside the kidney, they don't give the host any problems. If they move about inside the kidney, they can cause injury to the delicate tissues. Small stones can pass through the ureter in to the bladder, and out of the body through urethra smoothly without any knowledge of the host. However, if the stone is stuck anywhere in the passage causing a backup of urine, excruciating pain can result along with host of other emergencies. Immediate medical attention may be required at such a time.

CONGENITAL MALFORMATIONS OF KIDNEYS

Before birth the kidneys are located in the pelvic region and through gradual development move up to their normal position in the upper lumber region. In this process, some malfunctions occur:

****Ectopic kidneys*** are when they are out of normal place. A kidney may not reach its normal place or level. Or, it may cross to the opposite side of the body from which it originated. Ectopic kidneys are prone to infection.

****Solitary kidney***: Rarely a person is born with only one kidney; however, it is sufficient for the body to function.

****Horseshoe kidneys*** are those which paired, instead of being separated. They are linked at the lower end by a band,

****Polycystic kidneys*** have a tendency to run in the family. Both kidneys are studded with cysts. This disease progresses slowly and remains consistent with active life.

KIDNEY INFECTION

Bacteria can enter the body in many ways, and travel to the kidneys where it causes infection and inflammation. Bacteria can originate from the bladder, or in the surrounding tissues, and can travel through the blood stream and the lymphatic channels.

SYMPTOMS OF KIDNEY INFECTION

*Pain in the kidney region
*Fever, chills, nausea, vomiting, and changes in the formation of urine occur in chronic kidney infection
*Urine may contain pus, accompanied by a colony of micro-organisms, and a large number of white cells indicating that there is inflammation
*Frequent urination, or obstructive urination,
*Infected teeth can send infecting organisms in to the blood stream, which can reach kidneys
*High blood pressure
*Out of control stress

Early medical attention is required to clear up the infection, and neglect may result in kidney damage.

NEPHRITIS

Nephritis is a name fro several kidney diseases that are caused primarily by inflammation. It is the fine blood vessels of the filtering units of ***nephrons*** that are most commonly affected by ***nephritis.*** After the inflammation has set in, infection occurs. Salts of mercury and other metals can cause nephritis. Through the excretion process of kidneys which filters out harmful substances constantly can get scarred resulting in inflammation. Also, the blood vessels of kidneys can develop hardening of the arteries, which appropriately named as ***nephrosclerosis,*** resulting in restricted blood supply, high blood pressure and inflammation.

TUMORS OF THE KIDNEY

Tumors of the kidney may be benign or malignant. Malignant tumors are cancerous, and can travel to other parts of body.

The benign tumors are the fluid filled sacs, or cysts. They may produce a mass in patient's abdomen. Whereas malignant tumors develop in an active part of kidney, and occur only in one kidney, usually after the age 40.

SYMPTOMS OF MALIGNANT TURMOR

*Pain in one side of the body or the other.
*Bloody urine.
*Mass in the abdomen in the region of the kidney.

Symptoms may appear and disappear on a regular basis, and an immediate medical help is important.

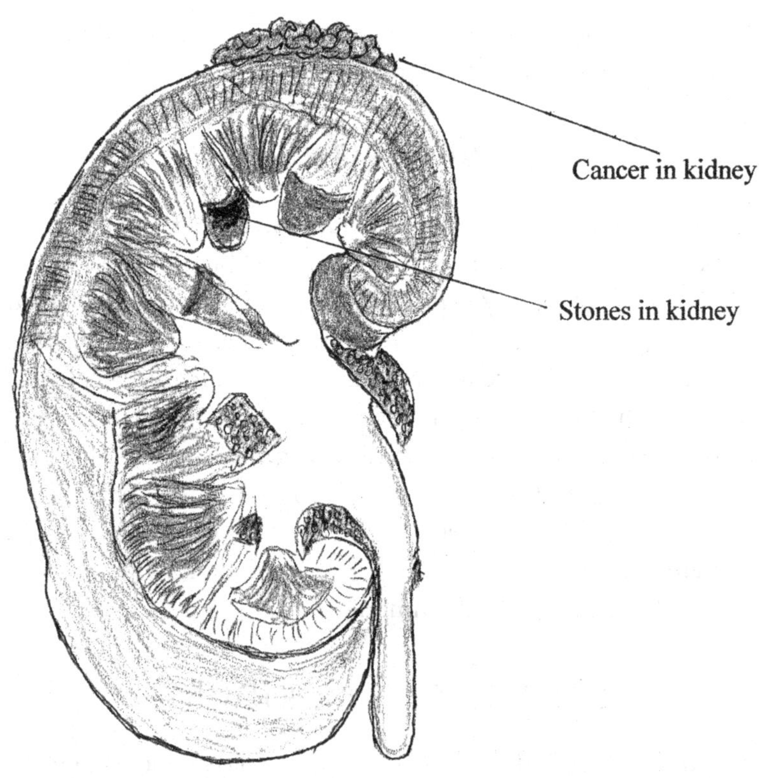

RENAL INSUFFICIENCY

It means that the kidneys are unable to filter all the wastes and toxins in the blood stream. Consequently, significant amounts of toxic substances remain in body, which are very harmful to the body. This condition can eventually poison the body, and cause death. The condition of poisoned body is called ***uremia.*** Un-excreted toxin can be deadly.

SYMPTOMS

Early stages of ***uremia*** are when the patient experiences headaches, muscle discomfort, itching, etc. In acute stage, the patient feels nausea and vomiting in addition to muscle discomfort, headache, and itching. The patient becomes drowsy, and reaches in to a coma and death. Therefore, it is important to consult the physician right away after experiencing any of the associated symptoms.

RECOMMENDATIONS

*Avoid tobacco smoke -- first and second hand

*Minimize the intake of foods containing ***cadmium*** found in various food products and also used industrially to manufacture rubber tires, paints, plastics, etc. Use cadmium-free paints, dyes, etc. Antique cookware may contain cadmium, so avoid cooking in them

*Discard all the old cans and bottles containing cleaning products, because they may be containing ***carbon tetrachloride*** which is highly toxic.

*Make sure that your shower room is ventilated, because

chloroform evaporates from chlorinated hot water, avoid using ***chloroform*** containing products.

*Avoid using cosmetics containing ***ethylene glycol*** which is also contained in antifreeze and brake fluids.

*Avoid using paint stripper, upholstery cleaners, spot removers, etc. Also, dry cleaned clothes, bags, etc. should be kept in an airy place for several hours before hanging them in the closet, because of ***tetrachloroethylene*** is used for dry cleaning purposes.

*Avoid using products containing ***oxalic acid*** like: heavy duty household cleaners, polishes, bleaching agents on the skin, eating rhubarb, etc.
*Minimize or eliminate alcohol and sugar intake
*Maintain a healthy weight
*Minimize the amount of starch, carbohydrates, and fats in your diet

*Avoid eating manufactured foods
*Avoid eating toxic foods.
*Minimize or eliminate stress in life
*Exercise regularly
*Maintain personal hygiene
*Visit your doctor immediately upon recognizing any symptoms

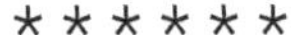

GALLBLADDER DISEASE

Gallbladder means storage container for bile. In Latin gall means bile. It is located just behind the liver. Gallbladder stores bile. It performs many functions and one of them to modify bile which is necessary to digest fat in the diet. Bile is a fluid consisting of bile salts, bile pigments, and other constituents. Gallbladder is saclike of about 3 inches long with a storage capacity of 1.7 fluid ounces of bile. It holds the bile, modifies it chemically, and makes it concentrated. At times, the contents of gallbladder get crystallized and become small stones which are commonly known as 'gallstones'. Every year, about 20 million new cases are reported with 650,000 hospitalized and about 500,000 are subjected to surgery in the United States.

Liver produces the bile which passes through a duct, known as 'common bile duct', and empties in to the small intestine where it interacts with fat in the food and digests it. Liver produces bile on a continuous basis, even though you don't eat fat all the time. Occasionally, bile enters the intestines when there is no fat to digest, it ends up getting wasted. When there is no fat in the intestine, the liver senses it and sends the bile to the gallbladder via the cystic duct which branches out of the common bile duct. If and when there happens to be excessive fat in the intestine for which the continuously produced bile seems insufficient, the liver sends the signal to the gallbladder which squirts out the required amount of bile through the cystic duct in to the intestine.

Bile salts and other constituents break down the fats in to tiny goblets, and eventually to an emulsion. The emulsification process makes the fats ready to be worked by pancreatic enzymes for the continuation of the digestion process. The stomach acids which are in the contents get buffered by the baking soda, contained in the bile, aids the digestion. Bile also carries the waste products from the liver, which makes it an essential tool for detoxification. The liver and gallbladder work hand-in-hand with each other on a continuous basis. When fatty food passes through the stomach in to the upper small intestine, a hormone called "***cholecystokinin***" (secreted in the small intestine) sends signal to the gallbladder to inject some bile in to the intestine. This also signals the liver to produce more bile to replace the spent bile.

PROBLEMS WITH GALLBLADDER

The gallbladder duct can get swollen causing reflux, thereby sending the bile back in to the gallbladder, which can result in spasm. Spasm can cause severe attacks of pain. Repeated pain attacks can scar the inner walls of the gallbladder and weaken its ability to function. Damage to the inner walls can cause inflammation of the gallbladder. The medical community calls this inflamed condition to be ***Cholecystitis.*** The lack of sufficient stimulus to the gallbladder can lead to back up, (low stomach acids and fat together stimulate the hormone which makes the gallbladder squeeze for the bile to excrete). Due to the lack of digestive enzymes, recurrent pain attacks can be experienced. Chronic gas, chronic belching, acute pain in the upper right of the abdomen, gallstones, severe pain after eating, especially fatty foods, nausea, are among the more noticeable bladder problems.

CAUSES

*Over weight, lack of exercise, skipping meals (especially breakfast).
*Food allergies which may be related to the consumption of cow's milk, eggs, wheat, coffee, pork, onions, etc can cause such problems.
*Constipation and a long transit time for food to pass from the mouth to the anus can cause bladder stones due to super saturated bile.
*Low levels of folic acids, fiber, and magnesium in the body cause bladder problems.
*Insufficient consumption of foods with E, B, and C vitamins can cause several problems. Gallstones can result due to lack of vitamin E.

*Overuse of refined sugar and carbohydrates inhibits the liver to make sufficient quantities of bile while, at the same time, saturating the bile with additional cholesterols.
*Hormone replacement therapy can cause gallbladder problems.
*Allergic complexes are formed and can affect various tissues adversely. Swelling in the gallbladder and bile duct can occur, and the flow of bile can be slowed down, or halted.
*For some unexplained reasons, women with fair skin are more likely to have gallbladder problems.

GALLSTONES & GALLBLADDER INFLAMMATION

It has been estimated that after the age 40, gallstones are present in 50% of women. 90% gallstones have no apparent symptoms. On an average, it takes about 10 years for the gallstones to develop. When there are gallstones, the most common symptom appears which is: severe pain in the upper right of the abdomen. This pain is a steady and gripping pain causing nausea. It is called '***biliary colic***', and the pain generally disappears after 1 to 2 hours. If the pain persists, the condition is called '***cholecystitis***'. Gallstones can block cystic duct, or common bile duct, or the pancreatic duct.

***Gallbladder inflammation (cholecystitis)** occurs when the bile sludge blocks the cystic duct. Acute pain is associated with this condition, which travels up to the right shoulder and other parts of the body. Breathing can become difficult and increases the pain. The pain is usually sudden and severe. The patient may develop fever. Diabetics are at more risk with this condition which often requires surgical intervention, or removal of the gallbladder.

***Chronic Cholecystitis** is a chronic inflammation of the gallbladder, and repeated attacks of pain in the upper right portion of the body including the right shoulder occur. This acute pain is accompanied by nausea, vomiting, and discomfort brought on by consumption of fatty meal. Gas, abdominal discomfort, nausea, chronic diarrhea may result under this acute and painful health condition. This severe and painful condition is primarily caused by a stone, may be several stones, in the gallbladder which loses its capacity and functionality almost completely. If stones cannot be removed then the gallbladder is surgically removed.

SYMPTOMS

*Yellow skin or jaundice.
*Fever, chills, vomiting, pain.
*Drop in blood pressure.
*Rapid heart beat.
*Dark urine.

*Loss of appetite.
*Metallic taste in the mouth.
*Bloating and general discomfort.
*Light colored stools, etc are the symptoms of cholangitis.

CAUSES OF GALLSTONE FORMATION

There are many theories outlining the causes of gallstones formation, however, some of the suspected causes are:

*Highly concentrated bile, resulting in the formation of stones.
*Excessive intake of fats, which may be increasing the concentration of bile.
*Liver disease, which may be causing inflammation.
*Gallbladder's inability to handle bile salts.
*Excessive calcium.
*Infection within, causing inflammation.

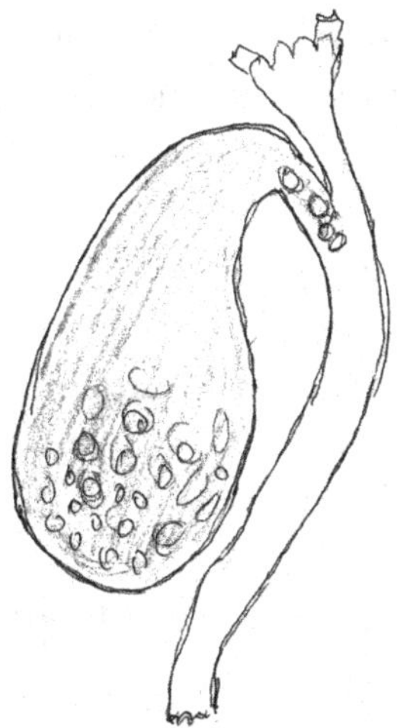

Gallstones blocking the cystic duct can cause inflammation of gallbladder

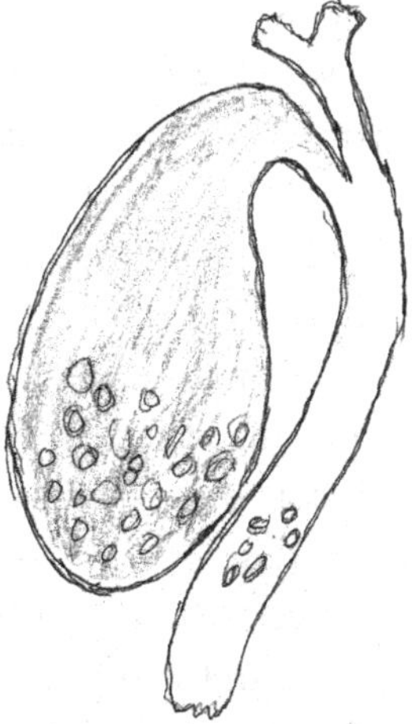

Gallstones in common bile duct blocking the flow of bile from gallbladder or liver to duodenum (can cause jaundice)

RECOMMENDATIONS

*High fiber and low fat diet should be adopted, because it will tend to keep the bile cholesterol in liquid form
*Small quantities of olive oil may lower your chances of developing gallstones. Gallstone problems are at minimum among people who consume olive oil regularly.
*Lecithin, the thickening agent in ice cream, found in soybeans, oatmeal, eggs, peanuts, cabbage, chocolate, and milk may help in eliminating the gallstone formation.
*Maintain your liver in good health, because if the liver fails to produce sufficient quantities of bile acids, gallstones can form even if you eat healthy.
*Use up the calcium in the body through regular exercise
*Regular checks by yourself will reveal if your face, skin, or eyes have some yellowish color, when it will be time to call your doctor.
*Taking Vitamin E which has been known to dissolve and prevent gallstones, Lecithin which is a great emulsifier of cholesterol and fat, and keeps it in liquid form; and Vitamin C which stimulates cholesterols to turn in to bile may help you to cope with gallstone problems.

*Drink more than 8 glasses of water every day.
*Lose weight if you happen to be over weight.
*Eliminate refined sugars, carbohydrates, and caffeine, or minimize them in your food.
*Eat as many fresh vegetables and fruits as you can afford.
*Exercising stimulates the bile production.
*Lower your blood cholesterol count because it will keep the bile liquid and prevent it from forming stones.

*Improve the bowel transit time by consuming high fiber diet

*Never skip meals. 12 hours or more without having food can cause gallbladder stones.
*Identify foods that you are allergic to, and eliminate them completely.
*Increase the intake of digestive enzymes.
*Avoid taking synthetic hormones.
*Eliminating anger, worrying, fear, and hatred related emotions from your thoughts will stop or reduce gallstone formation.

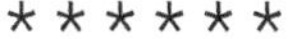

INTESTINAL DISEASES

Intestines are the real workshop where food is digested and reduced to nutritional components which are absorbed by the body and enter the blood stream. There are two many classifications of intestines—small and large.

SMALL INTESTINE is located in the center of abdominal cavity. It is about 22 ft or more long in coiled position. Its muscular walls knead food in segmented contractions, and shift food backward and forward. Most food products are absorbed in the small intestine. Food and water move along the intestine through peristaltic movements which are rhythmic constrictions of the intestine muscles. There are 3 sections of Small Intestine:

1. Duodenum, about 12 inches long and 1inch wide, begins at the stomach outlets
2. Jejunum, about 10 ft long
3. Ileum, about 12 ft long

Digestion of food is completed in the small intestine where the absorption of nutrients occurs through its mucosal lining. An estimated 5,000,000 small velvety fingerlike projections, called ***Villi,*** stud the intestinal wall. At the base of ***villi*** throughout the intestine there are about 35,000,000 glands discharge enzymes, mucus, and other intestinal juices.

LARGE INTESTINE is about 5 ft long and is divided in to 6 sections. It is responsible for the absorption of water and excretion of solid waste material. Waste material is moved forward along the length of intestine by rhythmic constriction of the intestinal muscles. Waste becomes solid because most of the water is removed by the intestine as it travels through it. The large intestine has been classified in several sections which are as follows:

1. Cecum
2. Ascending Colon
3. Transverse Colon
4. Descending Colon
5. Sigmoid Colon
6. Rectum

If the intestines are not working properly then it is concluded that various serious health conditions exist in the intestinal tract, which must be attended to immediately. While the intestines are processing the food content it takes a certain passage time, and the food contents become from green to brown. If the food content passed too quickly then ***Green Stool*** will appear and not brown. The appearance of ***Green Stool*** is indicative of laxative use, diarrhea, side effects of medication, ulcerative colitis, Crohn's disease, Irritable Bowel Syndrome (IBS), Celiac disease, cancer, Salmonella infection, or antibiotic reaction.

Crohn's disease could be the reason why intestines are not working properly. It is an ***Inflammatory Bowel Syndrome disease*** and not fatal. People having IBS may lead an active productive life for quite sometime until this disease starts producing other health problems associated with it. Mostly, the inflammation is confined to the lower part of the small intestine but it can affect any part of the digestive tract. It may affect severely or mildly to different people. Bleeding, fever, loss of weight, diarrhea, sores around the anal area, green stool, joint pain, fatigue, abdomen pain mostly in the lower right side, are some of the symptoms of this condition. It is also called **colitis** which is discussed in the following pages. (Also see Gastroenteritis)

It can block the intestine causing the patient to experience painful cramps, vomiting due to failure of food passing through the blockage, and a variety of problems associated with bladder, skin, vagina, inflammation in the eyes, kidney stones, gallstones, etc.

Constipation can disrupt the intestinal function entirely, which generally occurs when small amounts of dry and hard stool come out, and the bowel movement is fewer than 3 times per week. Constipation can cause painful bowel movement. Large piece of hard stool gets lodged in the rectum and blocks the passage. Watery stool can leak out around the lodged hard stool, which puts an excessive pressure on the rectum muscles repeatedly. This repeated pressure on the rectum muscles weakens them, thereby making it difficult to hold the stool. At this stage, constipation has created a disturbance of the functioning of intestines, which affects many other areas of the body.

It is a normal function of the intestine to absorb water and move the waste material forward, but when too much water is absorbed constipation occurs. Too much or more than normal amount of water is absorbed by the intestine when the intestine's muscles become slow and sluggish, meaning that food is moving too slowly and staying in the intestine too long. Some of the causes for food to travel in the intestine too slowly are: lack of exercise and dietary fiber, irritable bowel syndrome, pregnancy, old age, poor bowel habits, stopping or postponing need to go, lack of sufficient liquids, hemorrhoids, laxative abuse, Parkinson's disease, lupus, stroke, hormonal changes, etc.

Constipation can cause anal fissures, fecal incontinence, and numerous other health conditions most of which are the source of many life-threatening health conditions. Simple measures on daily basis can cure constipation. Adopting a regular schedule of physical exercise in association with plenty of water, vegetables, grains, fiber, beans, lentils, fruits, etc. should keep the bowel movements regular. More about this is mentioned in the following pages. (See also Constipation & Diverticulosis)

* * * * * *

IRRITABLE BOWEL SYNDROME

Irritable bowel syndrome (IBS) is associated with many adverse health conditions. IBS is functional bowel disorder of the gastro-intestinal tract which produces acute discomfort, abdominal pain, constipation, diarrhea, nausea, etc. It occurs in women more often than in men. 75% of all patients are women, and over 20% of world population suffers from it. IBS is also known as spastic colon, colitis, nervous stomach, and irritable colon at various stages. It causes abnormal stool frequency, lumpy hard to loose watery stool, passage of mucus, bloating, straining with sensation of urgency to evacuate, feeling incomplete evacuation, etc. The exact cause of IBS is unknown.

The most common foods that trigger IBS are meats from cows, pigs, chickens, goats, sheep, turkeys, deer, etc; dairy products, egg yolks, all fried foods, sandwich spreads, margarine, mayonnaise, fats, oils, chocolate, biscuits, pastries, pie crusts, coffee, carbonated water, artificial sweeteners, soda, artificial fats, MSG, etc.

SYMPTOMS

*Abnormal stool frequency
*Diarrhea and constipation, lumpy hard to loose watery stool, straining, urgency, feeling incomplete evacuation, passage of mucus, bloating, etc.

*Cramps in the stomach, and sometimes in other parts of body
*Inconsistent patterns of bowel movement
*Pain in the middle to the lower left side of your stomach

CAUSES

*Irritable bowel syndrome occurs when the movement of food becomes irregular which results from weak or irregular peristalsis (contractions of the intestines to move the food forward).
*Constipation caused by weakened intestinal muscles which move the food forward.
*Overeating overloads the system, and stops the food to move in a regular manner.
*High fat content in the food intake.
*Eating too fast, or eating at irregular intervals.
*Stress causes irritable bowel syndrome, among other serious health conditions.
*Antibiotics can affect the bowel habits because while killing the bad bacteria, good bacteria is also killed.
*Some prescription drugs containing morphine, codeine, other medication can interfere and alter the normal functions of the bowel and cause constipation.

RECOMMENDATIONS

*Take at least 30 grams of fiber in your food intake, each day.
*Give up smoking, and reduce the intake of foods containing caffeine.
*Exercise regularly, and include stomach exercises in your exercise schedule.
*Socialize and share your thoughts with others to release stress.

*Eat yogurt daily to populate good bacteria in the gut.
*Physician should be consulted for the proper diet intake. Avoiding high fat foods, caffeine, coffee, soda, alcohol, and all the gas forming foods like dairy products, beans, cabbage, cauliflower, etc should be helpful. The most effective dietary aid is fiber in oat bran, wheat bran, and psyllium which regulates the digestive system. It normalizes the bowel functions under both conditions—constipation, diarrhea. Also, it stabilizes the intestinal muscles, however, physician's advice is recommended.

******

INTESTINAL PARASITES

Parasite is an organ that resides in the body of another organism. Parasites live, feed, and colonize host's body. Intestinal cramps, fatigue, fever, diarrhea, and emptiness are the common indicators of hosting a colony of parasite in the body.

There are around 100 different types of parasites living in human body. Some are microscopic while others visible. Most parasites complete their life cycle in the hosts' body. They vary in sizes from $1/1000^{th}$ of a micron to 100 feet long whale tapeworms. They enter thc human body through food, water, sexual contact, nose, skin, mosquitoes, etc. While in the human body, these parasites eat the same food you eat, or they eat you.

CHARACTERISTICS

*People with intestinal parasite infection are weak, under nourished, infected with bacteria or fungi or virus, chemical and metal poisoning, etc.

*They can be present during any disease, in any person, and at any age.
*They steal the nutrition from your food, and secrete toxins (poop) in your body
*We provide the perfect environment for parasites to thrive through constipation, bad fats, junk foods, chemicals, sugars, and build up of fecal material on the colon wall

*Humans poison themselves with their own toxic waste and the toxic waste created by these creatures inside the body.
*Acceptable lab testing is available for only about 6% of these parasites of known varieties, with an accuracy of no more than 20%
*Cancer cases are afflicted with parasites which often lump together looking like tumor
*Depending upon the type of parasite, a female can lay 3,000 to 200,000 eggs per day in the body
*Most doctors, lab technicians, and lab staff members are not fully trained to recognize the associated symptoms of parasite presence in the body
*Out of about 3,200 varieties of parasites, some categories have been identified as major which are as follows:

MAJOR KNOWN PARASITES

Roundworms can produce 200,000 eggs per day, and more than 1 billion people are infected with it worldwide, making it the most common in the world. Symptoms are upper abdominal discomfort, eye pain, asthma, insomnia, rashes resulting from the waste products from worms. It can cause blockages in the intestinal tract, liver abscesses, appendicitis, loss of appetite, and hemorrhage during penetration of intestinal wall, pancreatic hemorrhage, food absorption deficiency, etc. It can grow to 15 inches long.

****Hookworm*** larvae can penetrate the skin, and young worms can cut through the intestinal wall to feed on your blood. Symptoms are iron deficiency, protein deficiency, loss of appetite, abdominal pain, skin irritation, dry skin and hair, edema, craving to smell or eat soil. It can cause mental dullness, delayed puberty, stunted growth, cardiac failure and death. It's about ½ inch long.

****Pine worms*** infect 1 in 5 children, worldwide. Symptoms are irritation of anus or vagina, itching, digestive disorders, nervousness, insomnia. Female worms can crawl out of the anus and lay about 15,000 eggs per day, and once airborne they can survive for 2 days in your living environment. About 500 million are infected with pineworms worldwide.

****Whipworms*** infect several hundred millions worldwide each year. Symptoms are blood in stools, weight loss, lower abdominal pain, bacterial infection, anemia, nausea, and hemorrhage during their entrance in to the intestinal wall. It is 1 to 2 inches long.

****Amoebae*** infect small intestine and colon, and releases enzymes that cause abscesses and ulcers. Also, they can travel to other organs including brain and the liver.

****Giardia*** is the most prevalent intestinal parasite found in the drinking water. Once in the body, they coat the intestinal walls which prevent nutrition absorption. Symptoms are light colored stools, abdominal cramps, gas, bloating, diarrhea, and weakness.

****Trichomonas Vaginalis*** are pathogens that reside in the vagina, and cause itching and burning sensations.

****Tapeworms (Cestodes)*** are of several kinds. Some of them are bladder tapeworms, pork tapeworms, dog tapeworms, broad fish tapeworms, rat tapeworms, etc. Broad fish tapeworms can grow up to 35 feet long and can live for 10 years inside the human body. Some tapeworms can lay up to 1 million eggs per day. Tapeworm Infection or ***Cestodiasis,*** although not dangerous in initial stages of infection must be removed just as soon as possible. If the condition remains untreated, these tapeworms can travel to other parts of the body including organs. They are a group of parasitic worms living in the intestinal tracts of many animals. They are segmented, and each segment is capable of producing eggs independent of the other. These eggs are dispersed through animal stools in almost every known environment. Some species of tapeworms find their way in to humans where they make their home.

Presence of tapeworms can be determined through stool testing, and other indicators happen to be fatigue, dizziness, loss of appetite, vomiting, loss of weight, Larva from the infected under cooked meats, insufficiently washed raw vegetables, etc. are the sources of tapeworm infection. Only doctors know how to treat this infection.

****Trematodes (Flukes)*** can cause severe diseases in the bladder, blood, liver, lungs, kidneys, intestines, etc. About 250 million people worldwide are infected with this parasite.

****Sperochetes*** are tiny organisms of spiral shape. They multiply in blood and the lymphatic system. They travel from lice, ticks, mites, fleas, flying insects and alike to humans. Their infection causes limes disease, infectious jaundice, sores, and ulcers. They are sophisticated and can fool body's immune system through posing as a part of the tissue. Once established in the human body, they can perforate the lungs, liver, intestines, blood circulatory system, etc.

PARASITIC DANGERS:

Once the parasites are in the body, they cause a host of problems. Beside eating up your food intake and therefore denying you of the much needed nutrition, they make their way in to the digestive system, liver, and other organs in the body. Parasites harm the body directly by being present inside the digestive system through robbing the body of nutrition, as well as through leaving toxins (poop) which are the by-products of their existence inside the body. Also, their harmful contribution does not end here; they colonize after embedding themselves within the intestinal lining, and spread. Parasites can travel to other organs, and also their toxins can reach many parts of the body without difficulty.

*1 in 4 people is infected with roundworm, worldwide.
*Predominantly, women host intestinal parasites.
*Parasites are picked up due to poor hygiene, during camping, traveling overseas, from pets, salad bars & buffets, tap water, institutional/group homes, etc.

Parasites interfere in the digestive enzyme, nutrients, and the digestive process causing major disruption of digestive system. Also, since their first priority is to survive, they can compromise body's immune system primarily to ensure their own safety and survival. The most challenging aspect of hosting parasites inside the body is to detect them, says Dr. Omar Amin of *Parasitology Center*, Tempe, Arizona. Parasites travel from one organ to another, remain active just for a day or two and then lay dormant for several days. This variable behavior on their part explains their absence from the stool sample. Dr. Amin suggests that several stool samples should be taken intermittently to determine the incidence of parasites in the body.

The relationship between the presence of ***Candida*** (yeast like fungi) and Parasites must be given full attention. Parasites eat away the nutritional resources upon which the good bacteria survive. In the absence of sufficient nutritional resources, the population of good (beneficial) bacteria is lowered. Under healthy conditions, the beneficial bacteria keep the population of Candida in check and consequently the population of Candida remains at an acceptable and harmless level. Reduced population of good (beneficial bacteria) allows Candida to suddenly jump in numbers. Yeast overgrowth or increased population of Candida causes 'attention disorder' and 'autism', according to Dr. William Shaw.

RECOMMENDATIONS

*Maintain healthy immune system
*Wash fruits and vegetables thoroughly after scratching protective wax if any
*Thoroughly cook meats, fish, and vegetables
*Drink clean water
*Eat yogurt daily to maintain the population of beneficial bacteria in the gut
*Wash your hands often
*Keep your home very clean
*Avoid walking barefoot on the warm and moist grass or soil.

*Avoid swimming in rivers, lakes, streams, etc.
*Make sure of your pets' cleanliness and health
*Avoid antibiotics if possible, but never overdo them
*Be extra cautious during traveling overseas
*Use cloves in your foods
*Clean your intestines through daily bowel movement
*Change the living environment of parasites. (Healthy cells and friendly bacteria in our body are ***Aerobic*** meaning they need oxygen to survive. Unhealthy cells, viruses, parasites, and pathogens are ***Anaerobic*** meaning they can only survive in non oxygenated environments)

* * * * * *

HEMORRHOIDS

Hemorrhoids are the varicose veins of the rectum, and develop in the lowest part of rectum and the anus. When the walls of veins stretch and become thin through swelling, called hemorrhoids, it becomes difficult to pass stool. It causes itching, burning, hurting, and bleeding of these swollen veins. There are externally visible and internal hemorrhoids.

> ****The externally visible hemorrhoids*** cause a lot of pain while passing stool, and even just sitting on the chair. Because of an ongoing pain and possibly some medication, some swelling occurs and some blood clots are formed in the area. Clotting and swelling may change color of hemorrhoids from red to purple. Some researchers call this condition to be ***thrombotic hemorrhoids***. If remained unhealed for a long time, an increased risk of infections, and some other diseases, including cancer, is possible.
>
> ****The internal hemorrhoids*** are in the deeper section of rectum, and are not visible. They are not painful, either, because there are fewer sensing nerves at that depth to communicate any pain to the brain. The internal hemorrhoids will give out some sensation of pain if they get out of control and for some reason they get enlarged and reach anus. With the physician's help, they can be pushed back. If they happen to be bleeding then the condition can be brought under control through proper medical help.

Some of the causes of hemorrhoids are: prolonged standing or sitting, weak veins, pregnancy, over weight, constipation, too much straining during bowel movement, etc. Excessive salt in the food causes fluid retention which results in swelling of all veins, including the ones that cause hemorrhoids.

RECOMMENDAIONS

*Vegetarian foods involving whole grains, vegetables, fruits, nuts, etc. *Additional fiber from Psyllium should be taken on daily basis.
*Stop using laxatives.
*Stop the consumption of manufactured and processed foods.
*Stop eating breads made with refined flours.
*Consume at least 4 oz of yogurt daily to maintain healthy gut environment.
*Develop and maintain toilet routine to avoid constipation and strain.

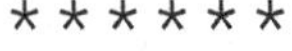

GASTROENTERITIS (INFLAMMATORY BOWEL SYNDROME)

Gastroenteritis is a general term for many kinds of intestinal infections, irritation, and inflammation. Intestinal inflammation can be caused by infection and non-infection. It is characterized by nausea, vomiting, diarrhea, abdominal cramps, low fever, and sometimes no fever. There are several conditions and related explanations under which this disease occurs and needs to be watched.

***ILEUS**

Ileus is the complete or partial non-mechanical blockage of small and/or large intestinal tract. There are two types of blockages—mechanical and non-mechanical.

Mechanical obstruction is when the bowel is physically blocked and the contents cannot pass the point of obstruction. This happens as a result of hernia, or due to the twisting of bowel on itself which is known as ***volvulus,*** or due to impacted feces, abnormal tissue growth, or the presence of foreign bodies in the intestines.

Non-mechanical obstruction is caused by muscular dysfunction inside the intestine, known as ***paralytic ileus***. It occurs because peristalsis stops. ***Peristalsis*** is the rhythmic muscular contraction that moves the contents through the bowel. The most prominent cause of this is an infection of membrane lining of the abdomen, also known as ***peritoneum***. It is a major cause of bowel obstruction in infants and children.

Reduction or disruption of blood supply to the abdomen is another cause of Ileus. Coping with bowel movement during and after the abdominal surgery can stop the peristalsis which can cause serious problems. People who have had abdominal surgery are more likely to experience Ileus. After the surgery, the condition of Ileus is temporary, but in some cases Ileus remains a challenge for a long time.

Ileus can be **caused** by stroke, kidney disease, heart disease, and lack of potassium. Stroke, heart disease, kidney disease, and lack of potassium can make bowel movement slow. Intestinal blockage does occur, primarily due to weakened peristalsis, and secondarily due to the lack of potassium and poor blood circulation.

The build up of gas, liquid, and content caused by ***Ileus*** must be relieved immediately. Usually, a tube is inserted through the nostrils in to the stomach and suction is applied to relieve the pressure and expansion. If the problem exists mainly in the large intestine, then a tube is passed through the anus of the patient to reach the large intestine to relieve the pressure. The patient is not allowed to eat or drink anything until the intestinal blockage is cleared. Fluids, sodium, chloride, and potassium are given intravenously.

*ILEITIS

Ileitis comes from Latin word '***ileum***' which means 'intestine', and the Greek word '***itis***' which means 'inflammation'. Ileum is the last of the three parts that make the small intestine. It is narrow and the longest part of the small intestine. It causes a sharp pain in the lower right side of the abdomen, can cause fever, swelling of the abdomen, constipation, difficulty in passing stool, and diarrhea. It can also cause loss of weight and anemia. ***Anemia*** is a condition when there is a deficiency of hemoglobin in the blood. ***Hemoglobin*** is a pigment that gives red color to the red blood cells which transport oxygen to cells in the body.

Often the **cause of Ileitis** is an ongoing irritation in the ileum, producing an abnormal reaction. It is difficult to identify what is causing the irritation. Various causes can be attributed to ileitis, and some of them may be: complications generated after an abdominal surgery, Crohn's disease, or infection of small intestine which can create inflammation. Sufficient rest and adequate nutritious food are generally the answers before the specific medications are prescribed, or surgical options are considered.

*PROCTITIS

Proctitis is also an inflammatory disease confined to the rectum. It is caused primarily by infection. Over use of laxatives, rectal injury, allergy, sexually transmitted diseases like Gonorrhea, Syphilis, Chlamydia, and the Herpes virus are the main causes of this inflammatory disease.

*COLITIS

Colitis is a general term for the inflammation disease which inflicts the colon and the rectum. The **symptoms** are excessive mucus coming out with the stool, blood with acute diarrhea, bowel movements during the night, fever, fatigue, weakness, pain in the joints, loss of weight, etc.

Mucus is secreted by mucous membrane which is a tissue lining on the inside of the intestinal walls. For a variety of reasons, irritable bowel syndrome causes increased secretion of mucus which comes out along with the stool. This health condition is known as ***Mucus Colitis*** which is caused by inflammation. Although this condition is harmless, nevertheless, it is a warning sign for something more serious to follow in the future. It needs to be attended to with the help of a physician.

On the other hand, ***Ulcerative Colitis*** is an acute inflammatory disease involving the colon and rectum with ulcers of various sizes. Blood with diarrhea are closely associated with this serious health condition. The exact cause is unknown for this disease, but several indicators point to allergies and hypersensitivity. Infection, arthritis, anemia, skin lesions, etc. are common among such patients.

CAUSES OF COLITIS

*Inflammation of the colon and rectum can result from most infections, viruses, toxins, and injuries. Parasites do invade our body and find home in the intestinal tract. Beside a variety of bacteria and viruses***, *amoeba*** often finds its way to enter human body. Amoeba produces poisons as a by product (poop), and these poisons tend to irritate the lining of the intestines. Similarly, other bacteria and viruses cause infection in the lining of the colon and cause Colitis.

*Antibiotics are often prescribed to treat infections caused by bacteria. If the antibiotics are taken more than 2 weeks in a row to kill the infection causing bad bacteria, it is most likely that this action has also killed good bacteria in the process. The good bacteria control another type of bacteria known as ***Clostridium Difficile***. When the good bacteria are killed by antibiotics and other medications, the population of the bad bacteria "***Clostridium Difficile***" gets out of control and increases. It introduces an irritating poison through its by-product (poop) to the colon lining, causing Colitis.

*Crohn's disease is another cause of Colitis, when any part of intestinal tract becomes inflamed. Also, if the supply of blood is decreased in the intestinal walls, Colitis can occur.

*Colitis can also occur if the blood vessels in the intestinal tract become narrower due to excessive blood cholesterols, or atherosclerosis, or due to old age.

* * * * * *

CROHN'S DISEASE

Crohn's disease is a chronic inflammation of the gastro-intestinal tract. Although this disease is mostly confined to the intestinal tract, it can appear anywhere between the mouth and the anus. It is also known as ***inflammatory gastro-intestinal disease***, **Regional Enteritis**, **ileitis**, **granulomatous**, and **ileocolitis**. Although the exact cause of this disease is unknown, it has been linked to the body's immune system response.

Inflammatory gastro-intestinal disease somehow disables the immune system which stops recognizing the good and friendly elements from the foreign invaders. Under the normal conditions, the immune system protects the body from the harmful substances and the foreign elements. But under these inflammatory conditions, the immune system fails to differentiate between the good and the bad, and treats all substances as foreign. This results in a continuous attack on all perceived foreign elements to protect the body. This condition is known as an ***overactive immune system response*** which gives way to chronic inflammation. When the immune system is always on the alert, it is called ***Auto Immune Disorder***, and is a serious and destructive health condition.

TYPES OF CROHN'S DISEASE

***Ileocolitis** is the most common form of inflammation in the intestinal tract. It affects the lowest third part of the small intestine, called **ileum** and the larger intestine, called **colon**.

***Ileitis** affects the ileum (the lowest third part of the small intestine).

***Gastro-Duodenal Crohn's Disease** is identified when there is inflammation in the stomach and a part of small intestine called **duodenum** which is the first portion of the small intestine.

***Jejunoileitis** is when there are spotty patches of inflammation on the middle portion of the small intestine, called **Jejunum.**

***Crohn's Granulomatous Colitis** affects the large intestine (Colon) only. Genes and the environmental factors play a role in the development of Crohn's disease which commonly occurs at the very end of the small intestine where it joins the large one (colon), however, it may occur anywhere in the digestive tract which runs from the mouth to the anus. This disease can occur at any age; however, most of the patients fall in to the age group of 15 to 35. Family history, cigarette smoking, and environmental factors mark this disease.

SYMPTOMS

The most prominent **symptoms** are:
*watery diarrhea, fever
*appearance and disappearance of flare ups
*belly cramps and pain
*blood in stools
*loss of appetite
*foul gas
*bad smelling stools
*pain in passing stools
*draining of pus from the rectal area
*skin rashes
*joint pain
*kidney stones
*deep vein thrombosis
*inflammation of gums and eyes.

RISK FACTORS

Crohn's disease patients have a higher risk of developing cancer of small intestine and the large one (colon). Also, severe problems may occur in the skin, vagina, bladder, besides developing abscesses, inflammation of the joints, lesions in the eyes, nodosum (red nodules under the skin), and ***erythema*** (the redness of the skin due to congestion of capillaries.

It is a life threatening health condition which requires

immediate medical attention. If the prescribed medication fails to bring satisfactory results, then the surgical removal of the diseased part of the intestine, or some other similar medical procedure may be required.

According to *Crohn's and Colitis Foundation of America*, as many as 70% of Crohn's disease patients will be required to undergo surgery at some time. Ironically, the surgical removal of the afflicted portion of the intestine does not cure this condition. Some patients end up with the need to remove the larger intestine (colon) entirely. Removal of the large intestine or a part of it is called **Colectomy.** The removal of both large intestine (colon) and rectum is called **Proctocolectomy**. After the surgery, a new pathway is created for the regular removal of body waste. The end of the small intestine is attached to an opening in the abdomen wall, and a pouch is attached. This pouch is worn outside the body like a soft belt underneath the clothing. Body's waste products are emptied out in this pouch which must be flushed out several times each day.

INTESTINAL VIRUSES

Viruses are something which is between a micro-organism and a complex molecule. They are neither an animal nor a plant. Viruses need a host, and cannot reproduce themselves. They are pieces of bad genetic code wrapped in protein, and cause disease by entering a host cell and controlling, replicating and destroying it before moving on to other cells. Body's immune system fights it, which causes inflammation. Inflammation caused by viruses in the intestinal tract is not uncommon among women, especially during later years. Many intestinal diseases are linked to intestinal inflammation which is a disease in itself.

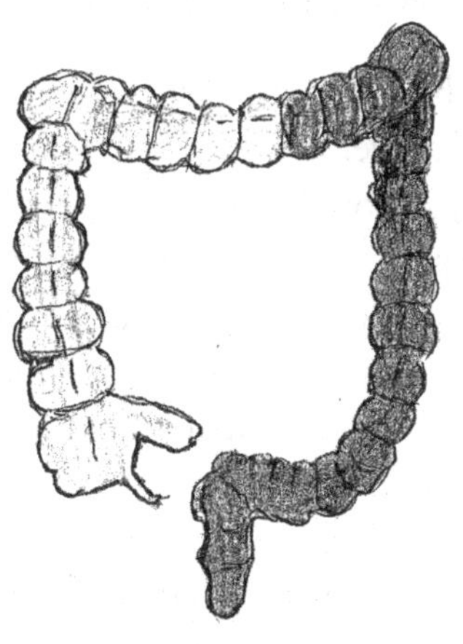

Inflamed, ulcerated section of colon and rectum in Colitis

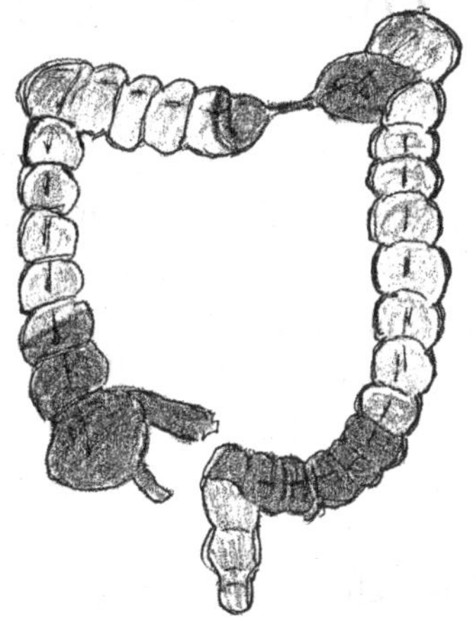

Inflamed, ulcerated, narrowed patches in Crohn's disease

RECOMMENDATIONS

*Taking about 30 gm of fiber each and every day.
*Eating yogurt every day to maintain the population of friendly bacteria.
*Maintaining regular exercise schedule.
*Drinking 12 glasses or more of water each day.
*Avoiding alcohol and tobacco.
*Avoiding refined and manufactured foods.
*Consuming at least 5 servings of vegetables and fruits of all varieties.
*Sleeping for at least 7 hours each day.
*Maintaining regularity in your bowel movement.
*Seeking advice from the doctor for any unusual symptoms.

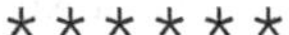

CONSTIPATION AND DIVERTICULOSIS

Constipation is when you experience hard and dried stools which are difficult and painful to pass. Bowel movement can become very difficult and injurious under constipated conditions. Most people in the world experience constipation periodically, some often. In the United States, about 400,000 new cases get hospitalized out of a total number of 3 million plus reported cases. There are probably 20 to 30 million Americans who suffer from constipation but find a quick solution to this health problem on their own.

Daily elimination or bowel movement is an important element of healthful life. It is also an important component of digestive system. Decreased frequency of bowel movement, or small and inadequate bowel movement (meaning that entire bowel is not getting emptied), or dried and hard stool indicate that the entire bowel is not emptying completely, Infrequent hard and dried stool is a sign that food is stuck in the intestinal tract and only a part of it is moving occasionally.

The stuck food in the intestinal tract puts an uneven pressure on the intestinal wall, tract, lining, and the cells. Additional burden is put on the intestines through straining and squeezing during bowel movement under constipated state, affecting the lower tissues of intestinal tract. Frequent or prolonged constipation weakens the intestine and its muscles. Prolonged constipation can affect the liver and the rest of the body.

A healthy lifestyle requires at least one elimination per day or more if possible. Food should travel fast through the intestines for good health. Longer travel time signals problems ahead. One bowel movement per day is the minimum, even though it may not empty the bowel completely which is still better than no bowel movement. Health problems emerge from constipation, poor or incomplete elimination, infrequent or a few days per weak bowel movement are signs of health problems which are initially experienced as headache, bloating, gas, allergies, anxieties, lack of mental energy, insomnia, depression, etc. Frequency, stool color, smell, presence or absences of undigested food, etc, are the rough indicators of the health condition of your intestines.

A good bowel movement is easy to pass, medium brown in color, full and round, without any blood, no excessive gas, not hard, not thin like ribbons or cables, and without bubbles. A bad bowel movement is when the stool is dried, hard, and difficult to pass, the stool is in small pieces having dark color, accompanied by excessive gas, bubbles, or blood, or mucus; in combination of soft and hard, and occasionally thin like cable, etc.

Constipation in a chronic stage is an extremely dangerous signal for a number of life threatening diseases and cancer. Chronic constipation occurs due to bad habits and carelessness. Long transit time for food to travel from the mouth to the anus is chronic constipation, and is indicative of:

*colitis,

*weakened colon walls

*hernia or diverticulosis

*hemorrhoids and rectal diseases caused by straining and stress

*colonization of unfriendly bacteria developed in the waste contents, and cancer producing substances that can penetrate the intestinal lining.

*Estrogen is affected by constipation which indirectly causes estrogen to get reabsorbed, thereby creating an environment of increased exposure to estrogen, which can cause:

-post menstrual syndrome

-endometriosis

-infertility

-breast cancer

-other cancers

-other hormones and their production are affected.

Excessive intestinal travel time of stomach contents to exit the body

*puts pressure on gallbladder, liver, and pancreas
*causes headaches and fatigue
*changes the gas pressure to reflux food backward damaging esophagus
*causes gas to rise upward irritating throat, gums, tongue, teeth,
*causes varicose veins to develop
*provides a scenario to develop lower back pain
*becomes a burden on the immune system
*causes bad breath

RECOMMENDATION

*Develop and maintain bowel movement habit, at least once a day.
*Exercise, movement, walking, staying active should be a part of daily life.
*Fiber in diet should be added without fail.
*Daily bowel movement will help keep estrogen levels in balance.
*Avoid dehydration by consuming plenty of liquids.
*Consume plenty of lubricants like olive oil, salad oils and seed oils, nuts which lubricate the mucous walls of the colon, and avoid hydrogenated and processed oils.

*Consume plenty of vegetables, fruits, cultured and fermented foods.
*Avoid or minimize foods without fiber like meats.
*Add olives, berries, figs, garlic, flaxseed, and mustard to your diet, which contain ***allicin***, which helps to stimulate muscles of the intestinal walls.

*Avoid using laxatives altogether.
*Take ***Inositol*** (part of vitamin B complex) which helps to stimulate the muscular wall of intestinal tract. Inositol is found in whole grains, citrus fruits, and brewers yeast.
*Take ***Pentothenic Acid*** (vitamin B-5) which helps patients after the surgery in intestinal functioning, as constipation can set in due to its insufficiency
*Consume ***yogurt*** daily to maintain friendly bacteria in the gut.

* * * * * *

DIVERTICULOSIS AND DIVERTICULITIS

Chronic constipation requires exertion and routine effort to pass the stool which has become dried, hard, and compacted. Frequently applied pressure on the colon wall creates some weak areas due to the regular strain to pass the stool out of the body. As a result of pressure, small sac-like pockets form on the inside of the colon wall. Initially, they are shapeless, but over time, they form a shape like a very small balloon bulging out from the inside of the colon wall. This condition is called ***diverticulosis,*** and is harmless if periodic clean up of these sacs take place. About 50% of people above 50 develop this due to aging and hereditary reasons. These pockets are quite common among women with chronic constipation. There are about 300,000 new cases of diverticulosis in America each year, and about 85,000 get disabled for quite some time. Diverticulosis is a very serious health condition, and could become a hub for several fatal diseases.

Feces get accumulated in these small pockets in the intestinal wall and become bacteria breeding spots. If these pockets filled with feces don't get cleared or emptied, they can cause inflammation, infection, and blockage of the colon, which is identified as

Diverticulitis. If unattended, diverticulitis causes bleeding, infection, perforation of the bowel, and cancer.

SYMPTOMS

*Acute pain in the lower abdomen, mostly on the left side.
*Chills, fever, nausea, stomach cramps.
*Constipation.
*Small and thin stools with diarrhea.
*Small pieces of stool and occasionally small round balls of stool appear.
*Persistent urge to empty the bowel, but nothing comes out.
*Feeling of incomplete bowel movement persists even after passing stool.
*Frequent visits to the toilet, but each time only small pieces of stool coming out.

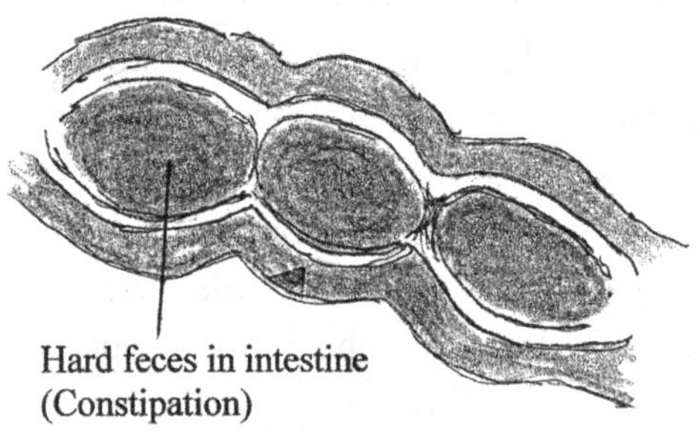

Hard feces in intestine
(Constipation)

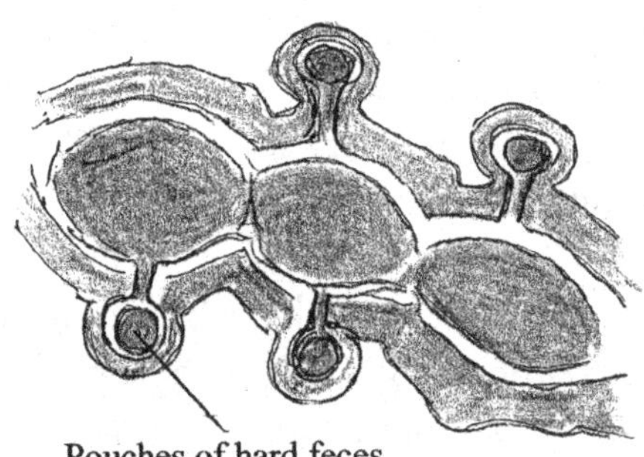

Pouches of hard feces
form in intestine
(Diverticulosis)

RECOMMENDATIONS

*Seek medical help immediately and get treated without delay.
*Once treated, maintain a healthy diet and lifestyle.
*Exercise regularly to stimulate bowel region of your body.
*Take plenty of fibrous foods, and drink lot of water without which fiber will not benefit.
*Make sure that your bowel movement is at least once a day, preferably twice a day.

*Incorporate raw garlic and onions in your daily diet because of their antibiotic attributes.
*Call your doctor at the slightest hint of inflammation, infection, constant pain, bleeding etc. which are the signs of ***diverticulitis.***
*Postpone eating solids until you feel your belly is cleared of waste matter.
*Eat yogurt daily to populate friendly bacteria in the gut.

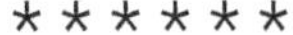

HERNIAS

Hernia is a condition that occurs when a tissue or an organ protrudes through the abdomen or any other weak spot in the body. Most hernias occur when a portion of intestine slips through a weak spot in the abdominal muscles. When this happens, a bulge will appear on the outside of the belly. One can feel it as well as see it. Hernia can appear in the groin, or the navel, or any other place where surgery has been performed previously. Hernias can occur through strenuous exercises when a weak spot in the abdomen opening gives away, and the portion of intestine or an organ loses the support of the abdominal muscle resulting in protrusion. Some hernias are present at birth, while others develop over a period of time; however, all occur due to some kind of weakness in the abdominal muscles. Hernias can appear in the diaphragm, esophagus, and other places in the body. Each year, there are about 400,000 women who suffer from hernia of one type or another, and more than 160,000 get hospitalized.

RISK FACTORS

*There are several weak areas in the abdominal muscles, and the groin happens to be the weakest**, both in women and men. In women, the suspending ligament of the womb that runs out from the abdominal cavity, and through a passageway, through the layers of abdominal muscles to its attachment at the front of the pelvis bone. In men, the cord which carries the pipeline from the testicles up to the abdominal cavity occupies a passageway, called the 'canal', between several layers of abdominal muscles in the groin. These passageways through the muscles are the weak spots.

*__Other weak spots are the navel and the pass__ageway where large blood vessels to the thigh leave the abdominal cavity.
*Also, muscles are somewhat weak in the **area of previous surgical operation.**

*Heavy weight lifting, and over exertion
*Excessive coughing, constipation
*Constipation
*Intestinal diseases
*pregnancy
*Over weight, etc. are some of the leading causes of hernias.

CLASSIFICATIONS OF HERNIA

****Reducible Hernia***: If the visible sac formed by hernia disappears when the patient lies down, the hernia is called reducible hernia.

****Incarcerated Hernia***: When the sac formed by hernia does not disappear then it is called incarcerated hernia**.** This means that the intestine is caught and can get twisted and become swollen.

****Strangulation Hernia***: The most dangerous condition is when the intestine is trapped in the sac and swells so tightly that stoppage of blood flow occurs. This condition is known as strangulation hernia and calls for emergency due to imminent danger of ***gangrene***. Physician's help must be sought immediately after any hernia occurrence.

****Femoral Hernia*** occurs when the intestine or bladder enters the canal (passageway through the abdominal muscles) carrying the femoral artery in to the upper thigh. Pregnant women and over weight women experience this kind of hernia.

****Umbilical Hernia***: When the small intestine protrudes and passes through the abdominal wall near the navel. Over weight women and women who have had several children before, and the newborns experience this kind of hernia.

****Inguinal Hernia***: When the intestine or bladder protrudes through the abdominal wall or to the inguinal canal in the groin, it is called inguinal hernia. About 80 percent of all hernias are inguinal hernia.

****Incisional Hernia***: When the intestine pushes through the abdominal wall at the site of previous abdominal surgery, it is called incisional hernia. This is common in elderly and over weight women.

****Hiatal Hernia***: Hiatus is an opening in the diaphragm. Diaphragm is the muscular partition that separates the abdomen and the chest. Starting from the throat, the esophagus passes through chest and reaches the upper part of the stomach. If the hiatus gets stretched and weakened, a part of stomach and/or a part of esophagus can get squeezed in to the chest cavity, like a small popped up balloon. Most people don't even know that they have hiatal hernia. They seem to be used to experiencing heartburn, bloating, shortness of breath, and some discomfort after meals. ***Heartburn*** occurs when the stomach's digestive juices make their way up in the esophagus, or in to the small popped up balloon squeezed in the chest cavity. There are a few classifications of hiatal hernias:

> *__*Sliding Hernia*__: When the upper portion of the stomach and the lower part of esophagus, connected to the stomach, move upward bringing both portions in to the chest cavity, the condition is identified as sliding hernia.
>
> *__*Para-Esophageal Hernia*__: If the stomach moves up through the hiatus and rests alongside the esophagus, it is called para-esophageal hernia.
>
> *__*Mixed Hernias*__: When features of both sliding hernia and para-esophageal hernia are present, it is called mixed hernias. When a portion of stomach or esophagus gets squeezed in to the hiatus, slow bleeding can result causing anemia. Also, hernia can get strangulated and so tightly constricted that the blood flow is cut off resulting in an emergency.

Most common is the ***sliding hernia*** and most women suffering from it are above 50 years of age. Like any other hernia, excessive weight lifting, over weight, pregnancy, constipation, over eating, insufficient exercise, lying down after eating or bending over, etc cause it.

RECOMMENDATIONS

*After 6 PM food intake should be minimum and not more than a snack.
*Bulk of the food should be eaten at breakfast and lunch.
*regular exercise regimen should be adopted.
*Active lifestyle should be adopted.

*Walking should be minimized after meals, if not completed avoided.
*Last meal of the day should be at least 4 hours before going to bed.

*Over exertion, over eating, excessive body weight, constipation should be eliminated.
*Minimum 5 servings of fruits and vegetables should be consumed each day.
*Drink plenty of water, that is, more than 8 glasses per day.
*Have a detailed dialogue with your doctor for any indications of discomfort.
*Eat your meals in small portions, chew thoroughly, and eat very slowly.
*Sleep with two pillows so that your head is raised above the level of stomach.

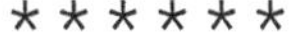

CHRONIC OBSTRUCTIVE PULMONARY DISEASE (COPD)

Chronic obstructive pulmonary disease is primarily a breathing difficulty which compels the patient to strain to bring air in and out of her lungs. Without air no one will survive more than a few minutes and, therefore, it becomes a straining, tiring, and fear generating exercise every minute of the day. It is a progressive disease, meaning that it gets worse progressively. It causes coughing, shortness of breath, wheezing, chest tightness, large amounts of mucus, etc. COPD is the 4th leading cause of death in America. It is projected to become 3rd leading cause of death worldwide in the year 2020 due to the increased environmental pollution.

When you breathe, the air goes down through the windpipe (***trachea***) in to the tubes of your lungs, called bronchial tubes or airways which are spread like branches of a tree. At the end of these branches are tiny air sacs, called ***alveoli***. In a healthy lung there are about 300 million air sacs in the lungs, which are responsible for delivering oxygen in the bloodstream and drawing out carbon dioxide waste. Alveoli sacs and the airways are quite elastic. Breathing in and out inflates and deflates the air sacs. Patients with COPD or chronic obstructive pulmonary disease experience less air flows in and out because of

*loss of elasticity in the airways and tiny sacs
*deterioration of walls separating the air sacs
*inflammation of walls which get thickened
*more mucus is made in the airways through clogging

It becomes a vicious cycle, and the disease continues to progress. In the United States, COPD includes emphysema and chronic obstructive bronchitis, and cause more than 68,000 deaths in women each year.

* * * * * *

EMPHYSEMA

Emphysema is potentially a fatal lung disease which typically causes chronic coughing, shortness of breath, and mucus build up. It is often caused by long time smoking, pollution, pre-existing asthma, and other lung diseases. When the thin walls of the tiny air sacs, ***alveoli***, get damaged, causing them to lose their shape and become floppy. The damage can also destroy the walls of air sacs leading them to become fewer and larger, instead of many small ones. Patients with emphysema are particularly vulnerable to pneumonia and bronchitis.

* * * * * *

CHRONIC OBSTRUCTIVE BRONCHITIS

When the lining of the airways is constantly irritated and inflamed, causes it to thicken and become hard. This results in the formation of mucus which clogs the airways making it difficult to breathe. Also, the patient is unable to cough it out or blow it out through the sinuses. It is a chronic condition and major cause of disability.

CAUSES

The most prominent cause for emphysema and bronchitis is tobacco smoking which breaks down the elastic fibers in the walls of air sacs which become prone to rupture. Tobacco smoke also weakens the walls of the lungs and makes them vulnerable to lung infections, and other serious conditions like bronchitis. A hair like cell '***cilia***' which is responsible for removing debris and mucus out of the lungs can get paralyzed by tobacco smoke. Damaged cilia become disabled to remove mucus which eventually accumulates and clogs the airways. Clogged airways are vulnerable to viruses, and bacteria infections. Clogged airways can also create conditions for asthma.

According to National Heart, Lung, & Blood Institute, most COPD patients have emphysema and bronchitis. COPD is a major cause of disability. 12 million Americans are currently diagnosed, and an equal number may be at the initial stages of this disease. The symptoms worsen progressively and limit patients' ability to carry out even the simple tasks. Most COPD patients are middle aged and older. There is no cure for it.

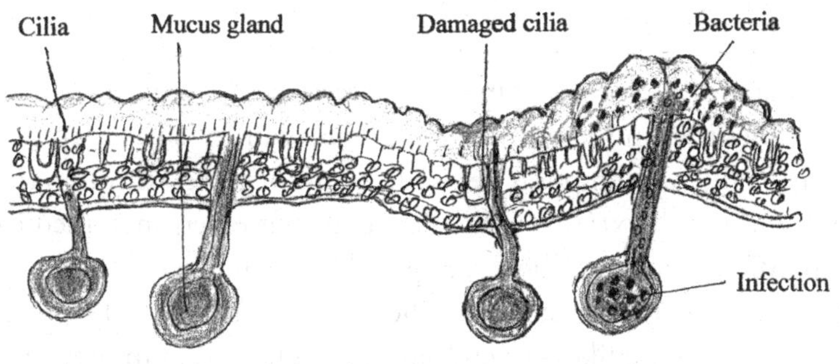

Normal bronchiole (airways) with healthy cilia to propel mucus upward to the throat

Inability of damaged cilia to propel mucus upward to the throat resulting in mucus build up causing infection (chronic bronchitis)

RECOMMENDATIONS

*Stop smoking, and stop being in the smoking environment
*Walk daily for at least an hour outside in fresh air.
*while standing up inhale and raise left arm high above your head, and bring the arm down slowly as you exhale. Do this exercise with your right hand also. This exercise should be repeated several times every day
*Get as much fresh air in to your lungs as possible through deep breathing exercises.
*Take a yoga class on breathing exercises, and learn to bring in nourishing oxygen to your lungs, or read a book on breathing exercises.
*Lie on your back on the floor, remain relaxed, and breathe so that your stomach inflates and deflates. Learn to breathe this way even during sleep
*Consult your doctor on regular basis if you experience any abnormalities in breathing.

******

ASTHMA

Asthma is a chronic respiratory disease, and is almost similar to bronchitis and emphysema. Some women suffer from it occasionally as a temporary episode, while others go through this frequently with extreme difficulty requiring emergency medical help. About 7 to 10 million young and old women experience this in America. Asthma takes a significant toll on the lives of women. Women are more likely to end up in the hospital than men, and it is more common among women than men.

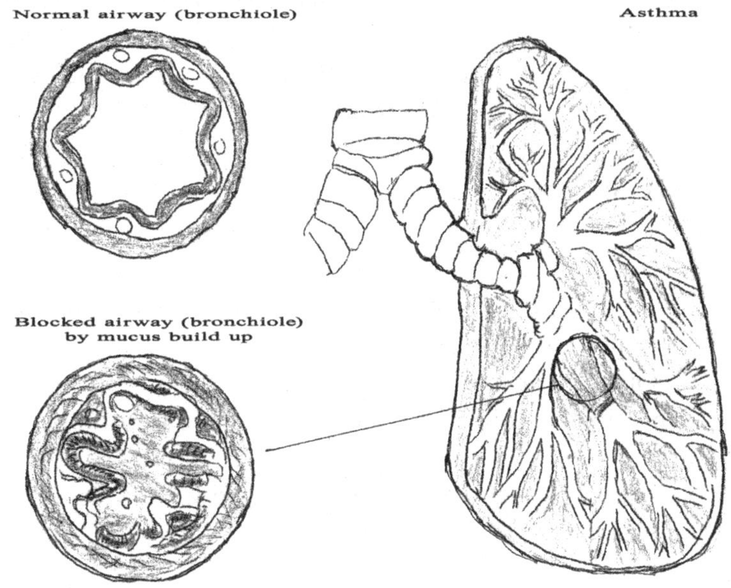

CAUSES

It is caused by several factors like: allergies (from dust, animal dander, pets, pollen, grass, tobacco smoke, mold, etc), bronchi, emphysema, lung infection, viral respiratory infection, etc. Allergies are the most common cause which is linked to release of ***histamines*** (amine compounds released in allergic reaction) and other body chemicals causing an allergic reaction which results in inflammation. Studies show that hereditary plays an important role in predisposing women to have allergic reaction to certain substances when inhaled.

Once the histamines released by the body's allergic reaction are in the bronchi, mucous membranes are stimulated and excessive mucus is secreted which makes the bronchi narrower. When exerted effort is made to inhale the air, mucus is pushed to fill the lung thereby causing blockage of the airway. Asthma is a very complex disease which is inheritable. There are several genes which make women susceptible to this disease, including genes on chromosome 5, 6, 11, 12 and 14. Much more research is on the way to shed more light on the exact role played by the genes in Asthma.

SYMPTOMS

*Difficulty in breathing.
*Insomnia and restlessness.
*Infrequent coughing with some phlegm.
*Gasping for air, and scared.
*Wheezing or whistling sound is heard when breathing.

Some researchers describe Asthma in two ways: extrinsic, and intrinsic

Extrinsic asthma is sensitive to allergies from the outside, which include mold, dust in the house, pollen, pets, feather pillows, cockroaches, sulfites in the food (as additives), etc. In most cases, extrinsic asthma develops during childhood and often accompanied by some genetic diseases like eczema and possibly some other.

Intrinsic asthma relates to internal factors, and is not linked to the allergies emanating outside. In most severe cases acute respiratory infection is the cause, however, there are a variety of other causes that create the condition of intrinsic asthma. This type of asthma is associated with and triggered by humidity, temperatures, exposure to noxious fumes, emotional stress, anxiety, fatigue, inhaling irritants, inadequate ventilation, etc.

RECOMMENDATIONS

*Maintain a complete account of the environment which

triggered the asthma attack, and consult your notes to determine the contributing factors which influenced the episode of asthma attack in the future.
*Maintain peace of mind, take the fears and long past traumas out of your mind.
*Practice meditation, believe in live and let live, learn to forgive, understand universal love, prepare yourself to deal with today and the future and leave behind the past.

*Monitor the variance in your lung capacity from time to time. If there is a significant change, you can take precautions by minimizing the severity of an oncoming asthma attack.
*Minimize, or eliminate sulfite containing foods like beer, wine, vinegar, pizza dough, lemon, apricots, apples, fresh shrimp, canned vegetables, molasses, instant potatoes, etc.
*Remove the dust from your living quarters regularly, and make it mold free.

*Live in a cockroach free house.
*Avoid using pillows and quilts stuffed with feathers.
*Stay away from tobacco smoke, and any other smoke and fumes.
*Let the fresh air in your living quarters every day, even during winter
*Visit the doctor immediately if experiencing acute breathing difficulties.

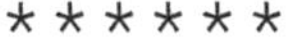

INFLUENZA (FLU)

Influenza is a dangerous viral infection which is extremely contagious. It occurs almost regularly during spring and winter. Influenza is similar to common cold in many ways. Both infect the upper respiratory system. Flu, a common usage for influenza, can appear in a matter of minutes and can make a sick person out of a healthy one. Flu can get in to the lungs. Flu can be fatal. Between 5% and 20% of the U.S population gets flu every year, and about 200,000 get hospitalized because of it. Approximately, 36.000 Americans die of Flu each year, and 700,000 worldwide. Millions die during flu pandemic.

The medical community has classified the influenza virus in to three categories; type A, B, and C.

> **Type A, influenza*** mutates constantly and develops new strains which make it difficult to take precautions by way of developing vaccines because the medical community cannot predict the type of new strain that will emerge. Consequently, vaccines developed earlier won't treat patients with the new viral strain.
>
> ***Type B influenza*** is linked to Reye's syndrome which has

mutation connections with other deadly viruses. Most influenza viruses jump from the animals to humans and back, mutating each time and creating entirely a new strain. Pigs or ***swine*** can catch ***avian*** (virus from birds including poultry) and human forms of viruses, and send a new strain back to humans. Avian virus which starts from the birds and poultry, and infects humans is always in a new strain of virus for which there is no cure or vaccine. Specific vaccines have to be developed to fight the new strain of the virus each time they appear, disregarding whether they are avian or swine originated.

SYMPTOMS

*Sore throat and chills.
*Dry cough.
*Muscle aches.
*General weakness.
*Sneezing and chest congestion.
*Headache.
*Fever between 101 degrees F to 102 degrees F, and sometime up to 106 degrees F.
*Follow your doctor's advice and get a Flu shot.

RECOMMENDATIONS

*Stop smoking tobacco and drinking alcohol because tobacco smoking and alcohol reduce the resistance levels in your body to fight any infection.
*Give wide berth to people who are coughing and sneezing.
*Avoid confined places like buses, airplanes, rooms full of people during the flu season.
*Maintain body warmth so that you can fight the invasion of flu virus.

*Greet other people without hugging or touching them during the flu season.
*Wash your hands after returning home from outside.
*Avoid sleeping in the room occupied by flu patients.

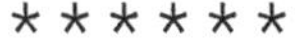

PNEUMONIA

Pneumonia is the inflammation of the lungs caused by a variety of viral, bacterial and fungal infections. It can also be caused by chemical exposure of the lungs. Lungs become congested with liquids. Most patients with pneumonia recover provided the symptoms are promptly recognized and treated. It's a dangerous disease and should not be taken lightly, because it can be from mild form to life threatening.

Inflammation in the lungs occurs when bacteria or viruses enter the airways, and get attacked by the protective white blood cells. The tiny air sacs of the lungs get inflamed and filled with liquid, leading to difficulties in breathing. The bacteria or viruses enter the body when its immune system is down due to tiredness, lack of sufficient nutrition, stress, etc, and the triggering of body's immune system to fight off the bacterial or viral attack further weakens the body, causing a major threat to the body. There are several kinds of pneumonia.

*__*Lobar Pneumonia*__ is called when the inflammation is limited to one lung or one lobe of one lung only.

*__*Bronco Pneumonia*__ is classified for the inflammation spreading from bronchi to one or both lungs.

***Double Pneumonia** is the term representing when both lungs are inflamed. This type of pneumonia can make breathing extremely difficult, and renders the patient exhausted and helpless.

***Viral Pneumonia** is caused by various organisms, and is generally mild and easily treatable.

Bacterial Pneumonia** is a very complex infection and life threatening. It is caused most commonly by ***Streptococcus. Average woman can get pneumonia from other people at work, in the train, bus, or in the shop, or anywhere. Once you get it, it can spread to other members of the household, or anyone in close proximity.

***Aspiration Pneumonia** develops when bacteria from the mouth or stomach enter the lungs, which generally happens during sleep, or during unconscious stage.

***Pneumocystis Pneumonia** (pulmonary infection caused by protozoan pneumocystis carinii) occurs when there is a good amount of weakness in the body's immune system. Patients with AIDS, Hodgkin's disease, and other diseases which suppress the immune system can develop this kind of pneumonia.

SYMPTOMS

*Coughing with blood.
*Restlessness.
*Fever.
*Muscle pain, fatigue, headache.
*Shortness of breath.
*Chills and shivers.

RISK FACTORS

While most common source of catching pneumonia is through close contact with other people, there is another very common source of catching pneumonia bacteria and viruses and that is from the **medical institutions**, mainly hospitals where patients spend some time to get well from other health conditions, and end up getting pneumonia.

Patients who are using **breathing machines** (mechanical ventilators), **patients with HIV/AIDS**, **patients with chronic pulmonary obstructive disease** (COPD), etc. are at great risk of developing pneumonia while in the hospital, or are being sent home from the hospital. These patients are vulnerable because their immune system is weakened, and it becomes easy for bacteria and viruses to enter the airways (bronchial pathways).

Pneumonia can cause additional diseases in the body through its occurrence. Breathing interference due to **lung inflammation** can cause infections to enter the blood stream and travel to other parts of the body very easily and quickly. Therefore, immediate medical help is an absolute must.

PLEURISY** can occur due to pneumonia. Pleurisy refers to the inflammation of membrane that surrounds the lungs and enables them to expand and contract smoothly. This double layered, lubricated, membrane (pleura***) is between the chest wall and the outer lining of lungs, which allows the lungs to inflate and deflate freely. Inflammation caused by pneumonia restricts this free movement, and constant rubbing takes place with every breath, cough, or sneeze. Also, fluids can accumulate here resulting acute difficulty and possibly pain in breathing. Lungs will not move even half the way, and the patient will not be able to draw a complete breath. Patient will experience a feeling of helplessness and nearness to death.

Just after pneumonia infection takes place, a small cavity is formed at the location of the infection. This **cavity can get abscessed**, which puts the patient at an additional risk. When you add abscess and pleurisy to pneumonia, all together make it almost impossible for the patient to breathe even half properly. This kind of barely breathing deprives the body of essential oxygen, which causes slow down in all body functions including the brain. If the condition persists and remains unhealed, the patient is most likely to go in to coma.

RECOMMENDATIONS

*Get a pneumonia shot with the help of your doctor.
*Avoid tobacco smoking, and the tobacco smoke environment, because it damages the ***"cilia"*** which is hair like and stops the irritants to enter the lungs
*Tobacco smoking, and tobacco smoke environment weakens your ability to fight viruses and bacteria that cause pneumonia.
*Avoid alcohol, because it weakens your immune system's ability to fight pneumonia, and many other infections.

*Be extra careful about your nutrition, and personal hygiene.
*Distance yourself from people who are coughing and sick through general observation.
*Minimize your exposure to the public places and crowds during weather changes, flu seasons, virus outbreaks, when you have cough and cold, when you are feeling weak, etc.
*Protect your body with adequate clothing, proper rest, and proper nutrition.

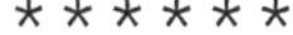

OSTEOPOROSIS, BONE FRACTURE, AND BONE CANCER

OSTEOPOROSIS

Osteoporosis is bone health condition which occurs when the bone loss outpaces the regeneration of new bone mass. In other words, more cells die and fewer new cells replace them in the bones. Consequently, bones become thin, a lot more porous, and fragile.

A decline in the production of sex hormones occurs when women are passing through the middle age. Sex hormones are essential to maintaining the continual process of bone tissues being broken down and replaced by new ones. When there is insufficient or minimal production of sex hormones, bones lose their mass, become thin and brittle, and more porous. After menopause, the estrogen levels in women's body fall rapidly which leads to thinning and weakening of bones, and is called 'Osteoporosis'.

The most prominent sign of osteoporosis is the loss of height. All women without exception lose their total height as they grow older, which is directly related to gradual deterioration of bones and decline in the bone density. Bone density decreases in the jaw bone which holds teeth, spine, hip, and shoulders first in most cases, and the process is so slow that it is hardly noticed on day to day basis. Dental problems, loss in the height measurements, gradual stoop in the neck and upper body frame, inability to reach higher in the kitchen cabinet, difficulty in maintaining upright position while standing or sitting, etc are the most common indicators of height loss due to low bone mass density.

Height loss in osteoporosis

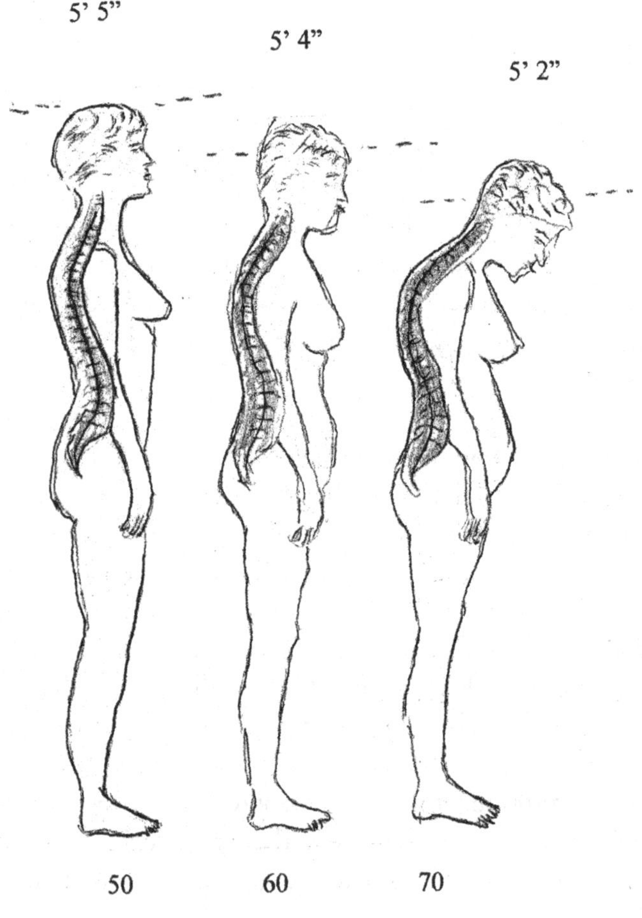

CAUSES OF BONE MASS REDUCTION

*Bone tissue consists of several minerals on the framework of collagen fibers. Majority of these minerals are calcium and phosphorus. Old tissues die and get replaced by the new ones. This process of continual regeneration slows down due to increased age, lack of sex hormones, overactive thyroid, poor functioning kidneys, smoking, etc, resulting in breakdown of the natural balance of tissue breakdown and renewal. The rate at which fibers, tissues, and minerals in the bones are broken down becomes far greater than the formation of new tissues in aging women. This causes weakening and thinning of bones, or bone mass reduction which in most women start right after the menopause.

*Additionally, the ability to absorb nutrients decreases in aging women. By consuming nutritious food and taking supplements, they believe they are meeting the nutritional requirements of the body when, in fact, less is being absorbed thereby unknowingly creating a deficiency.

*Bones are crucially important to hold the body muscles, to protect the organs by providing structure, and to store minerals including calcium. As women get old, a decline in the bone mass occurs naturally. Lack of sufficient calcium in the body compels it to dig it out of the bones, which results in the decline of bone mass. This condition leads to bone loss, makes them brittle and easy to break. Also, it takes much longer to heal from broken bones in women with osteoporosis.

RISK FACTORS

The bones become less dense and become much more porous.

The decreased density of bones makes them more likely to fracture, which can occur in the spine, hip, wrist, etc., and can deform the body skeleton including stooping disposition and loss of height. Women with osteoporosis are at a greater risk if they are suffering from other chronic or life threatening health conditions.

******

OSTEOMALACIA

Loss of calcium and phosphorus can lead to a somewhat similar condition to osteoporosis, called *osteomalacia*, which makes the bones much weaker and softer, and causes curvature of the legs. Patients become bow-legged. The direct cause of this condition is lack of vitamin-D beside calcium and phosphorus. Vitamin-D is obtained from food, sunshine on the skin, and from supplements which are vital to the absorption of calcium in the body.

******

FRACTURE OF THE FEMUR / HIP BONE

Femur is the thigh bone which is the largest, heaviest, and strongest bone in the body. The upper end of the thigh bone (***femur***) is the most common place where most fractures occur. Often people including the medical community call fracture in the upper thigh bone (femur) as "***hip fracture***" which is not the correct name because the pelvis bone, which is a part of the hip joint, is seldom broken.

Fixing fractures in the upper end of the thigh bone is a huge challenge because of the extreme difficulties in holding the broken bones in the right position for minimum 3 to 6 months. Since most of the patients who experience fractures of femur are above 60 years of age, the process and procedures of healing become equally perilous. An elderly patient is likely to catch bladder infection, pneumonia, etc. if she is subjected to stay in the hospital bed for 3 to 6 months, which can be life threatening. Today, under anesthesia big nails are used to join the fractures and the patient is able to use the 'walker' within a matter of few weeks.

Fractures in the higher end of ***femur*** (thigh bone) are much more difficult to set right because, in most cases, the only very small artery which nourishes the well rounded bone on the top gets torn along with the fracture that high up in the bone. If the well rounded head of the bone dies due to the lack of nourishment after the fracture, the round ball, or ***the hip,*** has to be replaced.

The prominent cause of the bone fracture at this portion of the thigh bone is the decreased angle (***coxa vara***) and/or increased angle (***coxa valga***) due to loss of bone mass and bones becoming more porous. Decreased and increased angles of the bone create an abnormal weight pressure on the portion of the joint where there was none before. The increased or decreased angle causes the impact of the body weight to shift to a different location. Weaker bones break when subjected to enormous body weight.

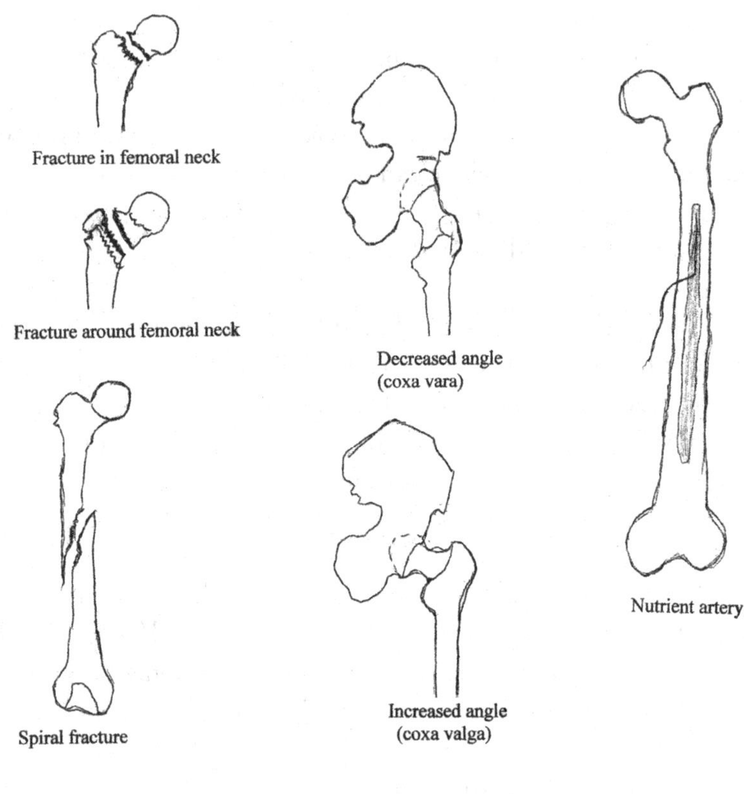

* * * * * *

HEALING OF BROKEN BONES

Bones are living tissues and grow with the rest of the body. They can repair themselves and continually go through the renewal process. When bones are broken or fractured, the surrounding blood vessels get torn or they bleed. Blood clots are formed. The blood supply is cut off and the affected blood cells die due to lack of oxygen and nutrients. The site becomes red and swollen. Germ fighting white blood cells, called ***phagocytes,*** rush to the area and start cleaning up the debris to prevent infection. At this very time, from the nearby bone a repair team of ***fiberblasts*** and ***osteoblasts*** is sent to repair and heal the broken bone. *Fiberblasts* cells produce ***collagen fiber*** which fills in the damaged area, while fibrous tissue made by the *osteoblasts* cells replaces the blood clot. This fibrous tissue is formed in to a callus. Blood vessels grow through this callus, and the *osteoblasts* cells start forming new tissue, and the process continues in repairing the bone for about two months by which time the missing bone will almost be replaced by new bone.

RECOMMENDATIONS

*Make every effort to increase bone density and bone mass in your body through adequate nutrition and exercise.
*Walk daily, and use your limbs by getting involved in every possible activity.
*Large amounts of calcium and phosphorus are needed for healthy bone growth, as are manganese, Vitamin A, Fluoride, Magnesium, Iron, Vitamin C, Vitamin D, Vitamin K and B 12 which should be included in your daily diet supplements.
*Get yourself checked by the doctor specializing in bones, on a regular basis.
*Drink plenty of water (more than 8 glasses); eat cheese and green leafy vegetables daily.

BONE CANCER

Bone cancer can be indigenous to the location on the bone, or has traveled from another part of the body. There are two broad categories of bone cancer.

PRIMARY BONE CANCER:

A cancerous tumor originating from within a particular bone has been described as primary cancer. Cancers that start from the bone are most likely to occur in young girls or young women. The primary cancer occurs in the long bones like thighs, has been classified as ***Osteo-sarcoma*** which causes swelling and severe pain. It can also break the bone. Under this category, if bone cancer occurs in breast bones, ribs, or pelvis, it is called ***chondro-sarcoma***. These cancers cause constant pain.

SECONDARY BONE CANCER

When cancer occurs elsewhere and spreads to the bone of a particular region in the body, it is called ***metastatic cancer***. Older women are more likely to experience this than the younger ones. Cancers in lungs, thyroid, breasts, and kidneys are the likeliest ones to spread to the bone. Most common areas of affliction are ribs, spine, pelvis, and the skull. Constant or nightly pain is the most common symptom of metastatic cancer.

******

OSTEOMYELITIS

This very painful type of bone inflammation is caused by infection of a bone, usually by bacteria. Osteomyelitis mostly occurs in women with weak immune system. The suspected bacteria may be ***Staphylococcus*** which causes the infection in the bone or bone marrow. Osteomyelitis related inflammation can also lead to bone cancer. Women on immunosuppressant medication and with tuberculosis are possible candidates for this type of cancer which occurs in pelvis, spine, and the bones of long limbs.

* * * * * *

OSTEITIS

Body continuously replaces old and worn out cells by new and healthy ones. So is the case with bones which are regularly repairing and renewing. Over time, hard deposits of earthly salts accumulate on the bone causing inflammation, pain, and bowing of bones. Many women after the age 50 suffer from the distorted shoulders, hands, legs, and other parts. This distortion is due to abnormality in the balance of bone formation which can lead to fractures easily. This bone abnormality, also known as ***Paget's Disease***, occurs mostly in pelvis, spine vertebrae, leg bones, and the skull.

When bone tissue breaks down and replaced rapidly by new but abnormal bone tissue, the outcome is a weakened, deformed or distorted bone. Women with distorted or deformed bones are generally in pain, and are at a high risk of bone fractures. Additionally, if the distorted or deformed bone ends up pressing a nerve, the patient will feel tingling sensation along with pain which will not go away. It may also cause numbness in the surrounding area and cause severe difficulties in functioning or using that part. Among several examples of deformed growth of some bones and their resultant affects on the neighboring nerves, the bone distortion in the skull may press the auditory nerve and cause loss of hearing.

There are other reasons which indirectly affect the weakening and fractures of bones and cause extreme pain, discomfort, and disability to women. Dislocation of bones, torn cartilages, bunions, bursitis, slipped disc (epiphysis), Perth's Disease, frozen shoulder, ***dysplasia*** (abnormal growth of bone) of the hip, osteoarthritis, rheumatoid arthritis, gout, tendonitis, ruptured tendons, carpel tunnel syndrome, muscular dystrophy, soft tissue inflammation, etc. are closely connected with the bones and nerves and affect the functionality and health of bones.

RECOMMENDATIONS

*Calcium containing green leafy vegetables and fruits should be consumed daily.
*Weight bearing exercises and walking should be a part of daily routine.
*Nutritional supplements and relative doses should be taken daily under doctor's guidance.

*Intakes of calcium, other minerals, and vitamin D should be sourced from nature rather than from manufactured products (vitamin D is available through exposure to sunshine).
*Young girls should peak their bone mass early in life, which will minimize the risk of developing osteoporosis later in life.

*Vitamin K and K 2 are important nutrients for the prevention of bone loss. Vitamin K 2 takes calcium from the blood and transport it to the bone, prevents destruction of cells which form new bones, maintains bone mass and in some cases increases it.

*Vitamin supplements should contain calcium, phosphorus, fluoride, magnesium, iron, manganese, Vitamins A, D, K, and B-12. ***(Vitamins A and C supports the manufacture of Collagen, the main bone protein, and keep Osteoblasts functioning). Bone making cells are called Osteoblasts.***

*65 mcg of Vitamin K should be taken each day, preferably from food sources like cabbage, kale, spinach, turnip greens, pine nuts, chestnuts, hazelnuts, etc. (for more information, please see the nutritional values pages in this book). If you are above 60 years of age, you should consider taking 90 mcg of Vitamin K each and every day.

It is quite challenging to cope with a health condition which requires much more nutrition after the age 60 when body's metabolism has already dropped considerably. Vitamin supplements in capsule form do not seem to work all the time, while you can consume only so much of green leafy vegetables and nuts each day. Try cooking large quantities of vegetables until they are reduced in size considerably, which will allow you to consume a lot of it. Also, if vitamin supplements have got to be taken then choose gel type over capsule ones.

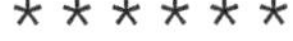

BLOOD POISONING (SEPTICEMIA)

Blood poisoning or septicemia occurs when bacteria from an infected wound in your body enters the bloodstream. Septicemia usually occurs to patients who have had recent surgical procedure, or some invasive treatment, or have a weak immune system. Women who fail to seek immediate medical attention find themselves in ***septic-shock*** which is a life threatening health condition. With the increase of invasive tests and surgical procedures, unfortunately the incidence of septicemia has also increased. If body's immune system fails to cope with the secondary infection after the test or surgery, and the bacteria continue to multiply, occurrence of septic shock becomes inevitable.

About 800,000 Americans experience acute blood poisoning or septic shock every year, and about 200,000 die from it. Women who are old, weak, with recent surgery, with weakened immune system, HIV/AIDS patients, with unhealed or slow healing wounds, and other infected wounds or injuries are most susceptible to getting blood poisoning. Bacteria such as ***hemolytic streptococci***, ***pneumococci***, and alike can manage to settle on a heart valve where they multiply and in no time can destroy it. Women with septic shock may have only 50% survival chance. The most common sources of blood poisoning are through:

BOTULISM

Botulism results from inadequately sterilized canned foods, or from cans which were not sealed properly and the foreign organisms entered and produced ***neurotoxins*** inside. It is caused by ***clostridium botulinum*** bacteria, found in the soil and the intestinal tracts of humans and animals. This toxin is a very potent one, and just a teaspoon of this toxin, if distributed, can kill several million people in a short time. Spoiled canned foods, foods in old or out of date or rusty, or leaky cans, improperly canned foods at home, etc. can be a source of botulinus toxins. There are differences in taste or smell from foods that have been contaminated.

GAS GANGRENE

Gas gangrene is a very painful and severe infection when muscles and subcutaneous tissues get filled with gas. It is caused by various species of ***clostridium*** bacteria which occurs in wounds that have been contaminated. Clostridium (bacteria) is commonly found in the soil and in the intestinal tracts of humans and other animals. It can occur to women who develop a wound during childbirth and the wound gets contaminated with feces.

TETANUS

The organism that causes tetanus is ***clostridium tetani*** which is found in the soil, streets, dirt, and the intestinal tracts of humans and most animals. These reproductive cells come to life only at times when insufficient or lack of oxygen occurs in their environment. They enter the body through wounds, dried or burnt skin, scratches, etc. and do not get noticed. Upon entering the body, these spores produce tetanus toxin which is very powerful and attacks the nerves. Generally, they take anywhere from a few days to several months to incubate. If they incubate rapidly, the symptoms of this poisoning are very severe, which may include irritability, restlessness, swallowing difficulties, stiff muscles, jaw muscles, etc. Tetanus poisoning produces progressively very painful condition and a horrible death.

OTHER CAUSES

*Secondary infection can occur in pneumonia patients, with any wound inside or outside the body, and cause blood poisoning. Most likely, the patient would experience septic shock from it.

*Septicemia can develop from eating unpasteurized dairy foods, including some soft cheeses that contain the bacterium ***listeria monocytogenes***.

*Eating raw seafood, especially raw oysters that have been infected with the bacterium ***vibrio vulnificus*** can lead to lethal septicemia.

*Women with liver disease, imbalance of iron, and weakened immune system are liable to experience the severest outcome of septicemia.

Bacteria from the infected wound on the body enter the bloodstream and infect it. Bacteria in the body poops in the body, and its poop is toxic beside its other destructive attributes. Presence of infection in the bloodstream triggers automatic response from the body's immune system to stop it, resulting in widespread inflammation. Widespread inflammation reduces the supply of blood to the tissues and organs .including the brain, resulting in dizziness. Inflammation causes formation of blood clots which impede adequate supply of oxygen to various parts of the body, and cause them to function at lower efficiency. If septicemia persists, body's immune system keeps on responding to the threat thereby causing chills, fever and inflammation.

SYMPTOMS

*Severe chills, loss of appetite, state of losing consciousness, dropping blood pressure.
*High fever, headache, nausea, heavy breathing, gasping for air.
*Dizziness, pounding of heart beat.
*Facial redness like a skin rash, etc. can be the signs of septic-shock.
*Restlessness, irritability.
*Stiffness of jaw muscles and some other muscles.

RISK FACTORS

*65 or older women with bacterial infection somewhere in the body are likely candidates.
*Women with recent surgical procedure are at high risk.
*HIV/AID patients are at high risk.
*Women who are in a medical facility, long term care, hospice, quarantine, etc can get it.
*Women with influenza or pneumonia are susceptible to blood poisoning.
*Diabetic women are at higher risk.

*Women working with poisons through occupation in labs and manufacturing facilities are more likely to get it.
*Eating raw seafood.
*Women involved in accidents, developing cuts and wounds in the street, dirt, and other unclean areas.

*Not washing hands with soap and water after touching or in close proximity of feces.
*Women with genetic predisposition to septicemia.

RECOMMENDATIONS

*Oral bleeding, especially dental, must be treated with the help of a physician.
*Boils, blisters, cuts, and other wounds must be given time, with or without medication, to heal completely.
*Patients after surgical procedures should make sure that the surgical wounds are completely healed before resuming activities involving the subjected limb.
*Medications prescribed to fight off the infection must be completed as directed by the physician.

*Adequate body hygiene must be maintained during and after the infection.
*Get vaccinated for influenza and pneumonia.
*Avoid coughing, spitting, and sneezing, environments.
*Take off your street shoes upon entering your home and wear house shoes if need to.
*Washing your hands frequently every day, especially after visiting the restroom and medical facilities.

*Getting anti-tetanus shot immediately after scratches, wounds, cuts, and bruises developed in unclean areas like, soil, streets, garden, restrooms, etc.
*Get immunized with protection against tetanus, and get a booster shot after any injury or wound thereafter.
*Visit your doctor immediately if a boil on your body becomes red or gets infected.

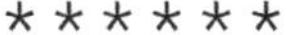

DIABETES MELLITUS

Diabetes is the 5th leading cause of death among women. Women are more likely to experience a diabetic coma than men. A diabetic coma can happen if a woman's diabetes is poorly controlled. Also, women are more prone to developing heart disease if they are diabetic than men.

The estimated number of diabetics in the USA is about 23,600,000. Also, there are about 17,900,000 who have been diagnosed. As the population ages, more and more diabetics may join these numbers unless proper health measures are taken.

Diabetes occurs when our body is incapable of making full use of the foods we eat, which are sugars, starches, and carbohydrates. The pancreas makes and releases ***insulin***, a hormone, to control the utilization of the available sugars, starches, and carbohydrates. When there is not enough supply of insulin, carbohydrates, starches, and sugars don't get absorbed by the body. Consequently, blood sugar remains in the system until it gets flushed out through the kidneys. Insufficient levels of insulin causing disorders of carbohydrates, sugar, and starch metabolism with increased urine production is called ***diabetes mellitus***. Diabetes has been classified in a few categories.

TYPE 1, DIABETES MELLITUS

Between 10 million to 20 million Americans are affected by this disease. ***Type 1, Diabetes*** called ***insulin dependant diabetes***, or ***juvenile diabetes***, results from shortage of insulin in the body. Beta Cells in Pancreas secrete ***insulin*** to correct high levels of glucose in the blood, and Alpha Cells secrete ***Glucagon*** which increases blood glucose if levels are low.

The shortage of insulin occurs when Beta Cells in Pancreas, which produce insulin, get destroyed or damaged by body's immune system which mistakenly marks them as foreign bodies. It is an auto-immune disorder which misidentifies the beta cells, and its cause may be rooted in inflammation or infection in the Pancreas. Damaged beta cells cannot release insulin, which leads to body cells not being able to take in glucose. Glucose remains in the blood thereby increasing the blood glucose levels.

Also, this damage may occur as a result of consuming sugars, carbohydrates, and fats consistently, and over exhausting pancreas through its non-stop production of insulin. Lack of glucose in the cells triggers the production of ***Glucagon*** produced by Alpha Cells in Pancreas, to increase the blood glucose if the levels are low. This increases the glucose levels in the blood even more. Too much glucose in the body but not enough in the cells is resulted.

Another reason for the shortage of insulin production by the pancreas may be attributed to birth defects. Pancreas may not be fully developed, or developed defectively, which produce insulin for a few years and then become increasingly inefficient. Pancreatic inefficiency or inability to produce enough insulin will lead young and older women to seek medical help.

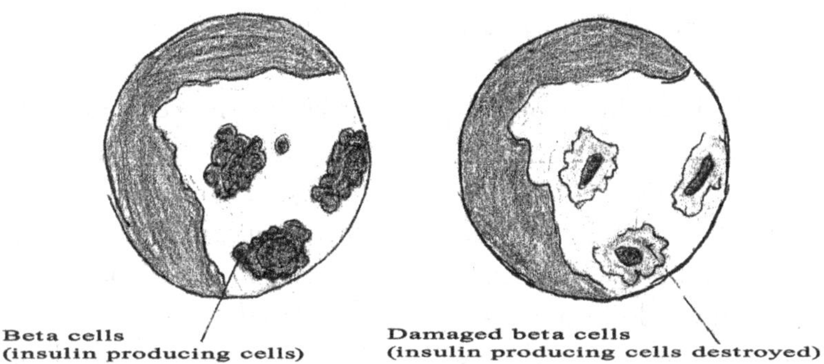

TYPE 2, DIABETES MELLITUS

Type 2, Diabetes results from the body's inability to process insulin effectively. About 90% of the diabetics have Type 2 diabetes. Sometimes it is called ***non insulin dependant diabetes***. It occurs when the body cells become resistant to the effects of insulin. For some unknown reasons the body cells fail to respond to insulin secreted by pancreas. Cells starve while the glucose and insulin are available outside of the cells. Cell receptors do not allow (or do not recognize the presence of) insulin to bind with them, and therefore glucose cannot be taken in to the cells.

Under normal conditions and when the cell receptors are normal, insulin will bind itself with the receptor on the surface of the cell. The binding of insulin with cell receptor sends signals to nucleus which triggers unlocking of the cell, and allows glucose to attach itself to the cell transporters which carry the glucose to the nucleus of the cell. Regular feeding of cell nucleus with glucose keeps the cell normal and healthy. On the other hand, when the cell receptors are damaged, weak, or dysfunctional; as in women with type-2 diabetes, insulin does not get attached to the cell receptors. This is due to dysfunctional, damaged, or weak condition of receptors who fail to recognize insulin and remain inactive.

When insulin does not get attached to the cell receptors, insulin floats in the bloodstream, and so does the glucose. Because the cell transporters get triggered only if the insulin binds with cell receptors, glucose does not get attached to the transporters which cannot take glucose to the cell nucleus. In other words, insulin must get attached to the cell receptors for glucose to get attached to the transporters without which no glucose will be picked up and fed to the cell nucleus. Without glucose, cells starve, weaken, and may die.

Type 2 diabetics lack the needed energy because the carbohydrates, starches, and sugars do not get adequately metabolized. If the body sugar drops to a very low level to fulfill the needs of your body, you can have an attack of ***hypoglycemia***, a serious health condition which can be corrected easily by recognizing the symptoms and consuming small quantities of sugar, carbohydrates and starches. In the absence of carbohydrates, starches, and sugars, body breaks down body fat for energy, which makes body highly acidic which is toxic and dangerous for the body. High toxicity can also occur when there is too much sugar in the body, called ***hyperglycemia***, and none in the cells. Once again, glucose starved body breaks down the fat and muscles for energy, making it acidic/toxic. A serious diabetic condition known as ***ketoacidosis*** occurs when ***ketones***, an even more toxic byproduct of accumulated acid/toxins, appear. Accumulation and concentration of highly toxic and acidic substances are life threatening.

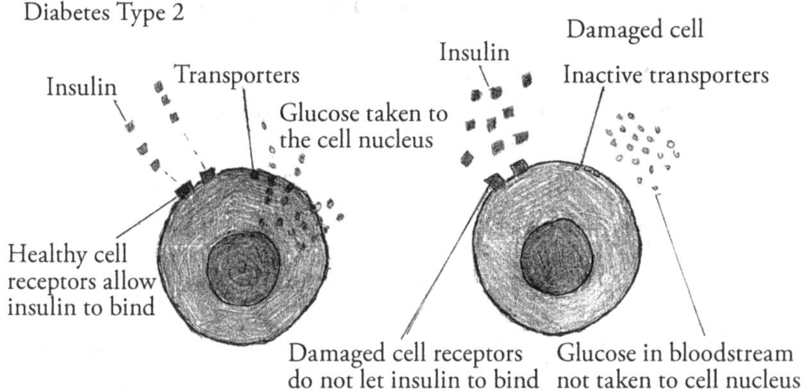

GESTATIONAL DIABETES

It occurs in pregnant women, and is more common among over weight and obese women. Some hormones produced by the ***placenta*** (an organ in the lining of uterus) during pregnancy have an anti-insulin effect, which increases the supply of glucose in the bloodstream, causing gestational diabetes. Fatigue, thirst, increased urination, yeast infection, bladder infection may occur. Under such circumstances the fetus grows larger and the delivery of the baby becomes difficult. Women with gestational diabetes are at increased risk of developing type 2, diabetes.

CYSTIC FIBROSIS RELATED DIABETES

This type of diabetes is induced by high doses of ***glucocorticoids*** (a kind of steroid hormones which raise the liver glycogen and blood sugar).

CONGENITAL DIABETES

This type of diabetes occurs due to the genetic defects which do not allow sufficient quantities of insulin secretion or none.

MATURITY ONSET DIABETES OF THE YOUNG (MODY)

This is another classification of diabetic condition with several sub categories, and is a subject of research these days. This type has several sub categories, and the most common is LADA (***latent autoimmune diabetes***), a slow developing autoimmune diabetes which is believed to have genetic overlap with type 1 and type 2 diabetes. It is believed that MODY is caused by 9 genes, and one needs to inherit only one copy of gene to displace the disorder. Some non-diabetic women carry MODY genes and while the symptom of diabetes may remain non existent, they may experience full fledged diabetes after the age of 50.

Statistics show that greatest susceptibility to diabetes for women is at 55 and men at 51. Married women are more likely to develop the disease than unmarried ones. A mother is more likely to develop this disease than one who never had any baby.

SYMPTOMS OF DIABETES

*Increased thirst and frequent urination (fluid is pulled from the tissues when access sugar builds up causing thirst which makes you drink, then you go to urinate).
*Increased hunger-(without sugar reaching the cells, muscles and organs get depleted of energy, which triggers hunger).
*Weight loss (without the ability to use glucose body taps

fuel stored in muscles and fat, resulting in loss of calories as excessive glucose is released in the urine).

*Fatigue (tiredness results when the body cells are deprived of sugar).
*Blurred vision (when the blood sugar is too high, fluids are pulled out of your eye lenses, which reduces the ability to focus clearly).
*Slow healing sores and frequent infections (Type 2 diabetes weakens your ability to heal and fight infection).
*Areas of darkened skin (signals insulin resistance).

EFFECTS OF DIABETES

**Cardiovascular diseases*: Women who have Type 2 diabetes are most likely candidates for developing cardiovascular diseases like stroke, high blood pressure, atherosclerosis, coronary artery disease, heart disease, dementia (Alzheimer's diseases), etc.

Risk for stroke and heart disease doubles with diabetes*: 75% with people with Type 2 diabetes die of stroke, heart disease, and cardiovascular diseases, according to *The American Heart Association*.

Nerve damage (neuropathy): Type 2 can damage the walls of capillaries, the tiny blood vessels that nourish your nerves, especially in the legs. It results in tingling, numbness, burning, or pains that start on the tips of the toes and gradually move up. It can cause reduced sense of feeling, and damage to the nerves which control digestion. Some patients suffer nausea, constipation, and diarrhea.

Ketoacidosis: Women should recognize the symptoms of ketoacidosis, which are excessive thirst, frequent urination, nausea, abdominal pain, and extreme weakness. If unattended, it can result in coma or death.

Kidney damage: Healthy kidneys through which waste is removed from your blood through a sophisticated and microscopic filtration system, a complex of about 1,000,000 *nephrons* in each kidney, are vital to your body's health. Diabetes can damage this filtering system causing kidney failure or irreversible kidney disease.

Damage to the eyes (retinopathy): Diabetes can damage the capillaries that supply blood to the retina which can affect vision. It is called retinopathy. Blindness, cataract, and glaucoma are strongly linked to diabetes.

Insulin imbalance: Too much insulin in the bloodstream can lead to brain damaging inflammation, and insufficient insulin can deprive the brain cells of nutrition.

Osteoporosis: Diabetes can lower your bone mineral density and cause an increased risk of osteoporosis.

Skin problems: Diabetes cause skin problems to occur. You can become a target for bacterial and fungal infections.

Foot condition: Damage to the nerves in your feet and / or inadequate blood flow to the feet, especially to the toes, can lead to very serious health conditions. Cuts, wounds, blisters can get infected easily, and also take much longer to heal. Additionally, gangrene can set, which can warrant the amputation of the infected toe, foot, or even leg.

Diabetic coma: Continuous high sugar in the urine, increased urination, fatigue, thirst, weight loss, vomiting, etc can lead to diabetic coma, which is a condition when the patient becomes half conscious with sweet odor in the breath. This can lead to death.

RECOMMENDATIONS:

*Monitor your blood sugar levels to maintain balance, which should be not too high and not too low, as determined by your physician.
*Lose excess weight just as soon as you can.
*Eat a healthy and balanced diet in small portions at a time.
*Regular exercising should become a part of your daily schedule.
*Blisters and sores should be attended to immediately with the help of a doctor.

*Small cuts, injuries, wounds, etc. should be seen by a doctor without delay.
*Toenails should be trimmed at least once a week with extreme care and without any cuts.
*Dry very shinny and thin skin on any part of your body should be cleaned with soap and water every night along with some doctor prescribed skin moisturizer or lotion.

*To improve blood circulation in your legs and feet perform daily exercises, and follow your doctor's advice in this regard. On your own, 1) raise your legs above the level of your heart and keep them there for several minutes, 2) lie down on the floor and place your legs on the edge of your bed or chair for a few minutes, and then bend them at the knees several times. These exercises will send the blood from your legs and feet to your heart for recycling.
*Never wear tight or ill fitting shoes, because blisters and corns can cause gangrene to diabetics.
*Report progress, changes, and the status of your health to your physician on a regular basis.

*Choose foods with a lower ***glycemic index*** which is the measurement of the effects of carbohydrates on glucose (sugar) levels in the blood. Lower number is better for you because it relates to the carbohydrates that breakdown slowly during the digestive process, thereby releasing glucose (sugar) at a slower rate in the bloodstream. Certain carbohydrates breakdown very fast, releasing glucose in the bloodstream rapidly, have been designated with higher index number, which also puts a pressure and burden on the body to produce sufficient quantities of insulin quickly. If the quantity of available insulin is insufficient, some glucose remains in the bloodstream causing diabetes.

Carbohydrates sources with low index numbers are the ones which breakdown slowly and release glucose at a slower rate, thereby allowing the body to produce adequate amounts of insulin with no burden on the body. In this way, all released glucose is fed to the cell nucleus at a slower and manageable pace. Consequently, no excess glucose remains in the bloodstream and, therefore, no diabetes occur. The following table indicates the approximate ***glycemic*** numbers for the most commonly consumed foods.

GLYCEMIC INDEX

Bread, white	95
Potato, baked	95
Rice, instant	90
Carrots, cooked	85
French fries	80
Pretzels	80
Cakes	80
Corn, corn flakes	75

Corn on the cob	75
Corn, canned or frozen	75
Bagels	75
Graham crackers	75
Cereals, sweetened	75
Rice, white	70
Taco shells	70
Spaghetti	60
Maltose	105 to 150
Glucose	100
Raisins	95
Honey, refined sugar	75
Watermelon	70
Apricots, dried	70
Pineapple	65
Ice cream	60
Banana, ripe	60

Foods that are least harmful or good for your

Cornmeal, brown rice	55
Wild rice	55
Popcorn, sweet potatoes	55
Whole wheat Pita bread	55
Yams	50
Green Peas	45
Beans	45
Beans, Pinto	40
Lima Beans	40
Beans, Kidney	30
Beans, Black	30

Butternut beans	30
Nuts, (most	30
Nuts, (some)	15
Artichokes	25
Asparagus	20
Tomatoes	15
Vegetables, green	15
Mango,	50
Kiwi	50
Pears	45
Apples, Plums	40
Peaches, Oranges	40
Yogurt with fruit	35
Milk, whole	35
Milk, skim	30
Cherries, grapefruit	25
Yogurt, plain	15

* * * * * *

ALZHEIMER'S DISEASE (DEMENTIA)

Brain aging happens when it loses or depletes cell reserves. After a certain age, and a serious illness, especially stroke, it is quite common to have cell depletion in the brain. Consequently, the population of dead cells increase, and when it is combined with the biological process which breaks down cells, tissues and molecules through oxidation, free radicals are created in the brain. Dead cells, tissues, and molecules are waste substances resulting from molecular degeneration, and need to be moved out of the brain for its healthy function. Vitamin E containing wheat germ mixed with fruits and vegetables, nuts, whole grains, yogurt, in varied combinations can help flush the waste out of the brain. Brain cells need nourishment on daily basis, and this feeding is crucial for the brain to function adequately, and to avoid senility prematurely.

About 100,000 brain cells die each day. To slow down the death rate and to maintain production of new cells each day requires protein feeding to the brain. As long as it is possible, we should see that the cells in our body keep on replicating and forming new ones each day. When cells stop replicating, or the replicating process slows down, we notice aging symptoms all over our body, including the slow down of the brain function. Depletion of our memory, energy, and ability to carry out day-to-day activities gradually take place as we enter the old age. It is a natural process for significant changes in our physical and mental life to take place as we grow older. However, when significant memory loss, mass confusion, acute speech and writing difficulties, etc take place due to some other factors, which cause our brain cells to fail us progressively, it directs our attention to some other health problem which is not related to the aging process. It's an abnormal condition known as ***Dementia*** whose cause is continued to be investigated. ***Alzheimer's disease is the most common type of dementia experienced by millions worldwide.***

Alzheimer's disease is named after a German physician, named Alois Alzheimer who in 1906 claimed that this disease is a brain disorder, quite different from the effects of old age. Since then, this brain disorder has been known as Alzheimer's disease. It's a progressive brain disease which is fatal, and so far no definite cause has been established for its occurrence.

It is the 7th leading cause of death in America, and more than 5 million Americans are living with it. Alzheimer's disease destroys brain cells causing all sorts of problems with memory, thinking, behavior, social life, etc.

Alzheimer's disease is the most prominent type of ***Dementia***, and accounts for 60% to 80% of all Dementia cases. Here is a list of types of Dementia:

*Alzheimer's disease
*Mild cognitive impairment (MCI)
*Vascular dementia
*Mixed dementia
*Parkinson's disease
*Frontotemporal dementia
*Creutzfeld-Jakob disease
*Normal pressure hydrocephalus

*Huntington's disease
*Wenicke Korsakoff syndrome

Our brains have about 100 billion ***neurons***, (nerve cells) and they communicate with each other in a network. It's a specialized and functional network whereby specific jobs have been assigned to a group of neurons. Some neurons are involved in 'thinking', 'learning, 'remembering', while others help us to 'see', 'hear', smell', etc. Yet, others tell our muscles when to move, and so on and so forth. In Alzheimer's disease and other types of Dementia, an increasing number of cells deteriorate and die. No specific cause has been found as yet, and the research continues.

It is different from Migraine, because there is no pain in Alzheimer's, and cells die at different sites of the brain. In migraine, the blood vessels get inflamed in one side of the brain and cause severe pain for several hours, or even several days. The following images will show the different areas of brain affected by Alzheimer's and migraine separately.

Researchers have been trying to identify the exact cause of Alzheimer's disease and coming up various explanations and markers. There are two suspects that may be linked to the Alzheimer's condition:

*Plaque build-up between the nerve-cells, and contain certain deposits of protein fragments called '**beta *amyloid***'.
*Tangles from inside the dying cells. ***Tangles*** are twisted fiber of a protein called '***tau***'.

Most people develop plaque and tangles as they age, but Alzheimer's disease patients develop a lot more than that. The important marker is that there is pattern in the formation of plaque and tangles which begin in the areas important to learning and memory, and then spreading to other regions. Some researchers believe that plaque and tangles tend to block the communication among the nerve cells and disrupt cell activity required for the cells to survive.

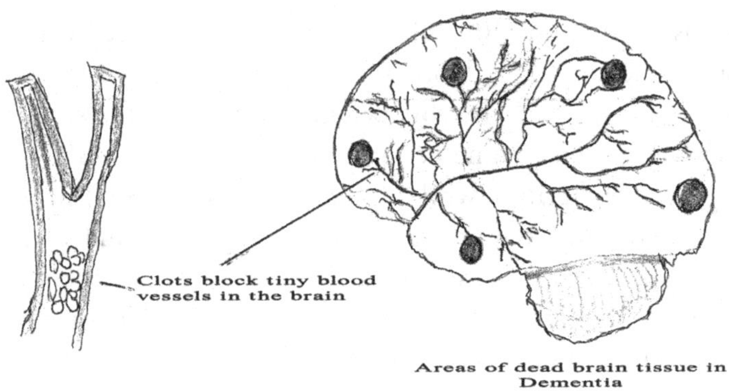

Alzheimer's disease

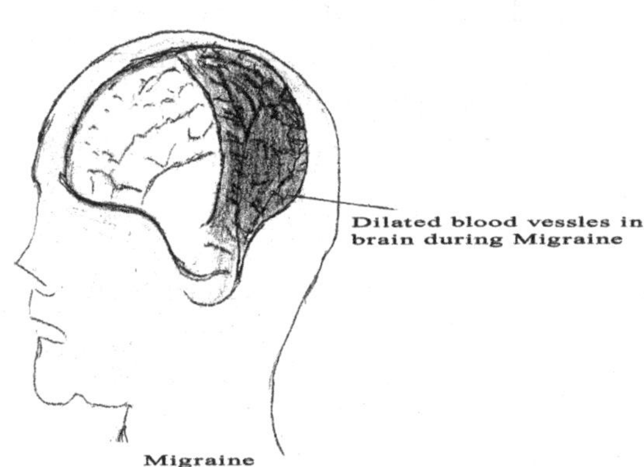

Migraine

RISK FACTORS

*Age 65 or older. Risk of getting Alzheimer's doubles every 5 years. After 85, the risk is 50%.
*Family history, hereditary, and the environment play significant roles in the occurrence of Alzheimer's disease.
*Diet of Animal meat and fatty foods.
*Genetics: 2 genes have been known to identify if a person is prone to Alzheimer's.

-Alzheimer's risk gene called ***apolipoprotein E-04 (APOE-e4)*** women with this gene may develop symptoms at younger age than usual. Scientists believe that there are many more like this one.
-Deterministic gene guarantees the infliction of this disease. Anyone who inherits this gene known as '***familial Alzheimer's disease'*** will get the Alzheimer's disease for sure.

*Head injury is another risk for Alzheimer's, because it can damage or destroy neurons, and contaminate their environment.

*Heart health is an important factor which cannot be ignored in the occurrence of this disease. Between 20% to 25% of the nutrients and oxygen is utilized by the brain which receives them through the blood supply. To ensure an obstruction free oxygen and nutrient filled blood supply is available to the brain, a healthy heart is necessary.

SYMPTOMS

*Forgetting recently learned information, names, events, dates, asking for the same info over and over again, etc.
*Difficulties in planning, problem solving, handling monthly bills, following recipes and procedures, etc.
*Marked changes in the mood and personality.
*Difficulties in completing familiar and even easy tasks at home or work.
*Confusion with place, locations, streets, time of the day, etc.

*Difficulties in understanding visual messages, images, pictures, spatial relationships, etc.

*Inability to make correct judgments, decisions, perceptions, etc.
*Problems with words, speech, writing, vocabulary, etc.
*The ability to retracing steps taken earlier, misplacing things, not finding every day things, etc.
*Avoiding people, social settings, workplace, and eventually withdrawing from them.

RECOMMENDATIONS

*Giving up eating animal meat and fatty foods.
*Regulate the intake of protein with your physician's help, and avoid too much accumulation of protein in the body at any given time.
*Eating lots of fruits, vegetables, and other heart healthy foods is just a starter. Efforts should be maintained to keep the heart running smoothly without any problems.
*Exercising regularly will help the patient physically as well as mentally.
*Even though social life is a constant challenge for Alzheimer's disease patients, a crusader's approach should be adopted, without shame, to socialize with others.
*Good mental health should over-ride any other emotion, including embarrassment and humiliation.

*Active participation in brain stimulating puzzles, games, and other recreations should be adopted.
*Avoiding tobacco smoke and its environment should be made essential.
*Every effort should be made not to cause any injury to the head.
*Vitamin E containing wheat germ mixed with fruits and vegetables, nuts, whole grains, yogurt, in varied combinations can help flush the waste out of the brain. Brain cells need

nourishment on daily basis, and this feeding is crucial for the brain to function adequately

*Incorporating ***turmeric powder*** in the preparation of meals should be tried, because Alzheimer's disease is almost non-existent in the countries where this spice is used in food preparations.

*Of course, personal physician should be consulted often.

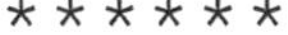

LAST WORD

In the preceding pages we have repeatedly noticed that the underlying causes are about the same in almost all the diseases and health conditions. Similarly, the recommendations encompassing the preventive measures were repeated in most cases. If all the killer or debilitating diseases are perceived from a distance, it can be determined that just a few changes in the lifestyle and the food intakes make the difference between a healthy woman and a patient. There are only a few problems with the '***diet and lifestyle***', which if corrected will reduce most women's risk of exposure to life threatening diseases. This statement is not without flaws. The diet and lifestyle can easily be controlled by women on their own, but controlling '**environmental exposure**', '**erroneous diagnostics**', '***unnecessary tests***', '**erroneous prognostics**', ***medical errors***, and '**genetic exposure**', are very difficult. The difficulties which lie outside the control of individuals can only be minimized or avoided for the time being, and we will explore the related options later. But first let us see what women can accomplish on their own by adhering to a diet and lifestyle which reduce, if not eliminate, the risks associated with deadly diseases.

DIET AND LIFESTYLE

You are what you eat' is an old adage which has been around for a long time, and is so appealing. There are some basics that women will be able to include in their diet in a very convenient way. If most of these foods are not already in your regular diet then make an effort to incorporate them just as soon as you can. It does take some time to get used to new foods and begin to develop a taste for them. Similarly, the body takes its own time to get accustomed to deriving nutrition from a new source, accepting new kinds of nutrition, its metabolism and absorption.

****Foods*** that you may wish to incorporate in your weekly diet schedule:

-beans, lentils, peas, seeds
-nuts (all kinds), fresh fruits, dried fruits, dried seeds
-green, yellow, purple, and red vegetables, with emphasis on dark green leafy vegetables
-red grapes, red grape juice, one glass of red wine (if not under any medical restriction)
-green, or black tea, or some coffee
-tofu and tofu products
-onions, garlic, chili peppers ginger, turmeric, cumin, parsley, mint, coriander greens (cilantro), dried condiment mixture containing Pomegranet seeds and rock salt, ginger, lemons, lime, vinegar, and various herbs of your choice
-some dark chocolate,
-low fat cheeses, low fat milk, yogurt, yogurt shakes,
-maintain a healthy balance of Omega 6 and Omega 3 in your diet. Both are available with varying degrees in vegetable sources like: olive oil, tofu, soy milk, berries, peas, flaxseeds, beans, walnuts, etc.
-vegetable oils and salad oils containing

polyunsaturated and monounsaturated fats, and without arachidonic acids, (Trans Fatty Acids) should be in your diet
-flaxseed meal, oatmeal, wheat germ, whole wheat flour, brown rice,
-some eggs, some fish, and some lean meats (if absolutely necessary)
-plenty of water, that is, more than 8 glasses each day

{{There are plenty of healthy diet programs in the marketplace, including diet plans based on genes and blood types. Dr. Peter D'Adamo has shown some broad categories of people with certain genes to thrive on a specific diet. He has broadly classified human genes in categories like: hunter, gatherer, teacher, explorer, warrior, and nomad, etc with inter-relation with various types of blood types, and recommends specific foods consumed by humans at various stages of development (hunter, gatherer, teacher, explorer etc). In a few cases, it may prove to be workable, but so is the case with every diet ever been developed. Also, Dr. D'Adamo basis his diet plan on the most recent stages of human development, which constitutes a very small portion of our genetic makeup which, in reality, dates back to millions of years, and not just a few hundred thousand years.

Each human is unique and not exactly similar to the other. It is possible to have two humans with the similar fingerprints, or eyeball prints, though extremely rare yet possible, but it is impossible to have two humans with exactly similar genes, or genetic makeup. Therefore, genetic diet may work for a few and not for most, which makes it just like any other diet plan.

Therefore, creating a universal diet plan for certain segments of genotypes, or blood types, will not prove to be functional. You should eat what is available, you can afford, you like, you can digest, suites your lifestyle, and doesn't make you sick, but in moderation to very small portions. Buying only the right kind of foods is a good start, because you will see them in your kitchen and will end up using them in the food preparations of your choice, taste, affordability, etc. Consult the nutritional charts and nutritional contents of foods, and incorporate them in your diet to obtain the maximum benefits. Each individual is different with different background, genes, growth environment, and health condition, social needs, economic status, nutritional needs and food choice, so make your own menu and manage your own diet. You are the best person to bring the required changes to respond to your changing health condition and several other influencing factors in your daily life.}}

***Develop a good Metabolism.** For the day to day function of our body, we need the chemical energy for which we need to consume calories from the food sources. To convert the food calories in to chemical energy, we require a metabolic process. A good metabolism converts the food calories in to chemical energy efficiently and with a minimum effort. Eating a lot does not mean a high metabolism. Inadequate diets, improper breathing and poor digestion are very common reasons for poor metabolism.

Pull yourself out of the depressed state of mind** which can cause digestive problems, poor breathing, and lack of activities, etc which in turn can lead to insufficient supply of oxygen in the body, which is necessary to burn the food we eat. ***Depression also causes lack of circulation, diabetes, and associated diseases. Mind affects our body in just about every way. A depressed mind can influence the immune system (through sending stress signals to the body) thereby, causing problems associated with our nervous system, stomach, metabolism, etc and causes auto-immune disorders. Therefore, healthy and adequate diets with happy state of mind are essential for all women.

***Adopt a disposition of pious, just, peaceful, reliable, sincere, caring, loving, well meaning, polite, helpful, respectful, courteous, friendly with no enemies and no fears, without greed, hatred, and jealousy; and a spiritually higher person.** Once these attributes have been ingrained in you, many of the killer diseases may not appear at all or will have much less potency which can be easily cured.

Psychological traits have a great influence on body's immune system, and are linked to the affliction of many diseases. Emotions of anger, fear, worry, retribution, etc. are interpreted by the brain as stress signals or an imminent danger to the body. This triggers body's immune system or the protection system to guard the body. Constant stress, fear, anger, etc. tires out body's immune system by keeping it on the alert all the time, causing wide spread inflammation, and its subsequent inability to protect the body from the foreign invaders. When the body is on constant alert, the immune system goes out of control and fails to recognize friend from a foe, called the ***auto-immune syndrome,*** it starts attacking the healthy tissue as well and cause wide spread inflammation. Wide spread inflammation causes many life-threatening diseases. Therefore, it is healthy to maintain a peaceful and spiritually high disposition at least most of the time.

Adopt meditation in your daily schedule. Meditation will improve your immune system, and concentrating ability.

****Minimize consuming animal protein.*** We should eat preferably just the right amount of total protein (preferably from non-meat sources) that our body requires to make and repair tissues. The excess amount of protein is used as energy source by our body. You don't need excess amounts of protein, you need just enough to maintain and repair tissues. Over and above this required amount of protein will be used as body fuel. Protein molecules are big and quite complicated, and their digestion requires much more work out than carbohydrates and fats. Vegetarian diet can easily meet this requirement. High quality protein from animal flesh is associated with lots of fat, toxins, hormones, and parasites which can be unhealthy for the body, can cause many diseases, and is not required. Adopt the vegetarian food option for your daily food intake.

Energy output from consuming protein is less efficient as compared to that of other nutrients. Additionally, protein fuel does not burn clean. Protein contains nitrogen, and after metabolism it leaves a toxic nitrogenous residue which eventually goes to the liver where it turns to urea which, in turn is flushed out by the kidneys. It is a burdensome task for the liver and kidneys to process this toxin, which can weaken the immune system temporarily.

Whereas, carbohydrates and fats are composed of carbon, hydrogen, and oxygen, and after metabolism carbon dioxide and water are left. Energy from carbohydrates and fats, in moderation, is efficient, and considerably easy to burn, without negative after affects. Adopting a vegetarian diet can prove to be beneficial in the long run.

About 30 to 40 grams of protein per day depending on the body weight, age, and health condition is more than enough, and this can easily be obtained from vegetarian diet. Roughly, 7 grams of protein for every one kilogram of your body weight is more than enough for your daily consumption, that is, if you are young and very active. For women above 50, a much lesser dose of protein will be sufficient, because their body's wear and tear is much lower along with the reduced strenuous activities. Also, the lesser doses of protein will have a much lesser burden on the liver and kidneys to flush out the unused protein.

Protein from animal source should be minimized if not completely eliminated because

1) There are plenty of other sources of protein from non-meat sources;
2) there is no need to kill other animals for food,
3) Various diseases, hormones, toxins, and parasites may be contained in the meat, which can be transferred to human body,
4) Humans have left behind the "hunters and gatherers" stage in the process of evolution,
5) The animals being eaten and the humans are genetically close to each other. Animals are genetic cousins of humans. By changing a bunch of genes in the human genetic code, one can get the genetic code of several animals, and
6) The scenario of ***"one animal is eating another"*** does not make humans as a highly developed and advanced species.

****Adopt an exercise routine*** you will be able to perform most of your life. Strenuous exercises take their toll on the body, are difficult or impossible to perform on daily basis or regularly. Walking, biking, aerobics, yoga, or simple daily household chores are some of the exercises you can do in to the old age.

****Maintain regular schedule*** for resting, bedtime, social, mealtime, pastime, and meditation hours.

* ***Make sure that you get at least 7 hours sleep*** every night. Lack of sufficient sleep sends stress signals to the body which responds to it by releasing stress hormones, primarily ***cortisol,*** and sugar in the bloodstream thereby causing inflammation and high brain activity. Inflammation causes several diseases including heart disease, and high brain activity leads to its higher consumption of sugar, alerts immune systems responses, suppresses the digestive system, generates fear, affects just about every function of the body including moods and behavior.

DANGERS TO AVOID

***_Avoiding exposure to toxins_**, chemical pollution, etc. in the environment should become an important part of life style. Toxins and pollution can damage DNA which contains the vital and crucial information for repairing and mending the body. Aged women have weaker immune system than the younger ones and, therefore, it becomes much more important for the aged to avoid toxins and pollution.

***_Avoiding radiation_** from various sources should be considered seriously. We all need to be careful of radiation however, for a senior or a patient; it becomes much more important to avoid lengthy exposure to it. Ultra-violet rays have big wave length, and regularly sustained exposure to it can damage the DNA in the skin cells, and can also cause cataracts in the eyes. So just be careful whether you are a patient or not; it can happen to anyone.

There is another kind of ***radiation*** which has short wave length. This radiation is highly dangerous. It is the same radiation which emanates from a nuclear explosion and operating x-ray machines. This radiation of short wave length can knock electrons from DNA, and make them ionized which can give room to a host of other health problems, besides damaging the cells. Higher doses of radiation of short wave length, which includes all kinds of x-rays, can damage the immune system. Avoid unnecessary and excessive exposure to x-rays, as much as you can manage to. Also, avoid its accumulative effects.

Plenty of fruits and vegetables in the daily diet may block the chemical reaction that leads to the injury to DNA, but there is no guarantee. However, do make an effort to avoid heating pads, electric blankets, electric clocks, computer screens, and damaged microwave ovens, Microwave foods only in ceramics or glass utensils. Never use plastic containers in the microwave ovens, because use of plastic can introduce foreign molecules in the food. Do not live near the Microwave Transmitter, or in the path of Military Communication site.

****Avoid dehydration*** by drinking a lot of water on daily basis. To remain healthy or to get better, women should avoid ***dehydration*** which can be especially dangerous for older women. When we are young, our bodies contain about 90% of water, and this water content of our bodies keeps falling in percentage as we grow older. Among elderly persons water content falls to 60%, or even lower. Water acts as an insulator. When it is cold outside, water content in our body acts like an insulator, thereby maintaining the suitable body temperature, and when it is hot outside, water keeps us relatively cool by maintaining the suitable temperature of the body.

Dehydration can cause thickening of blood, insufficient blood circulation, and kidney problems like: infections, stones, etc. For stroke and heart patients dehydration can be deadly, because thick blood will increase the possibilities of the formation of large blood clots which will not be able to pass through the blood vessels of the brain and heart. To combat various dehydration related kidney problems, patients have to take medication which, in turn, puts extra burden on kidneys, because the medication will end up passing through the kidneys. Also, lack of water makes the blood much thicker than normal. Kidneys are subjected to enormous pressure to pass thick blood which has to pass through the kidneys to get rid of body waste, which can result in darker urine. Urine should be pale yellow, and if it is darker then personal physician must be consulted.

In order to avoid all these unpleasant experiences and uncertainty of the outcome of such a condition, women are advised to drink a lot of water which can keep their system flushed on daily basis. Also ***dehydration*** causes accumulation of metals and toxins in the body. Eliminating or minimizing the concentration of metals and toxins in your body will help you live a healthier and longer life.

Even though it is impossible to live in this world without constantly getting exposed to various metals and toxins, the least we can do is to minimize such exposure. You will be surprised to learn how dangerous our cooking pots, water pipes, paints, sprays, etc, are. Knowing the dangers alone will help you to effectively deal with the related health problems.

Avoiding poor blood circulation** is the first step to improve your health. To prudently deal with ever existing day to day challenges, beside eating right and avoiding obvious dangers, women require a good ***circulation of blood in the body. Blood circulates adequately when the blood vessels are free of fat and cholesterol, and regular ***exercise*** which stimulate the muscles, joints, bones, organs, glands, etc. Some women get their exercise from the daily household and / or menial work routine of the day, while others need to do it through spending time in playing sports, in gymnasium, walking, or running, etc. Besides improving the blood circulation, exercise brings physical and mental relief from stress, worries, anger, unresolved difficult situations, etc.

The primary purpose of physical exercise should be to restore and increase blood circulation. The type, frequency, and the duration of any adopted exercising method should be something you enjoy and can continue deep in to the old age. Walking and swimming fall in this category, however, there may be other choices more preferable to some women.

Poor blood circulation is the cause of many life threatening health conditions. Blood circulation is responsible to move nutrients and wastes to and from cells. Also, blood circulation stabilizes the body temperature and the pH level. In general, ***poor blood circulation***

causes leg ulcers, boils, muscle cramps, blood clots, hemorrhoids, varicose veins, memory loss, cardiovascular diseases, etc. The most prominent ***risk factors of poor blood circulation*** are insufficient quantity of fluids in the body, dehydration, reduced volume of urine, high levels of chemicals in the urine, high levels of uric acid, calcium, and phosphate are present in the urine, urinary infection, stone formation, obesity, family history, high bowel absorption of calcium, over active parathyroid glands in the neck, etc.

Preventing Poor Blood Circulation:

*Drink more than 8 glasses of water beside other liquids.

*Eat green leafy vegetables, fruits, whole grains, legumes, etc.

*Consume limited amounts of sugar, salt, alcohol, caffeine, protein, and dairy products.

*Eliminate white flour, process foods, packaged foods, refined foods, etc.

*Drink lemonades made from real lemons with limited sugar.

*Adopt a routine of walking, aerobics, light sports, etc on daily basis.

*Lie down on the floor and put your feet up on the edge of the bed or a chair, and after a few minutes bend your legs at the knees several times. The repeated action will send the blood from your feet and legs to your heart for recycling, and consequently improve the blood circulation over a period of time.

****Avoiding wrinkles and dryness in the skin*** should be important for all women. Wrinkles and dryness allow foreign elements to enter the body and cause diseases which may or may not show any symptoms around the place of their entry point. Moisturizing the skin with baby oil is soothing, easy, and beneficial. Wrinkles in the skin appear as women age due to the decline in the supply of ***Collagen*** in our body, or through dryness of the skin. In essence,

Collagen is a protein available in the skin, bone, cartilage, tendon, and teeth. It forms fibrous connective tissue between the cells. Decline in the supply of this protein causes the connective tissue to weaken or get broken, resulting in the formation of wrinkles at the site of damage. Collagen is found in Brewer's yeast, peanuts, dried peas, nuts, sunflower and sesame seeds, wheat germ, olives, avocados, and some other plant foods. Once these plant foods are combined with fruits and vegetables containing vitamin C, the beneficial effects and the absorption of Collagen are enhanced tremendously.

Also, the combination of these foods can improve cardiovascular function, cerebral circulation, protection against cellular degeneration of neurons in the brain, and in general optimal functioning of the brain. ***Collagen*** in combination with ***vitamin C*** is healthful for the skin which is the largest organ of the body. With this combination tightness of skin will be experienced, and the roughness of the skin will increasingly diminish over a period of time. Combine ***Collagen*** containing foods with Vitamin C containing foods which are citrus fruits, strawberries, tomatoes, broccoli, Brussels sprouts, cabbage, green peppers, potatoes, sweet potatoes, kale, collards, mustard greens, etc. Practice various combinations of foods according to your taste, availability, and circumstances.

****Avoid premature brain aging*** by occupying yourself with creative activities and keeping busy. Premature brain aging starts when it loses or depletes cell reserves during and after a serious health condition. After a certain age, and a serious illness, especially stroke, it is quite common to have cell depletion in the brain. The population of dead cells increase, and when it is combined with the biological process which breaks down the cells, tissues and molecules through oxidation, free radicals are created in the brain. Dead cells, tissues, and molecules are waste substances resulting from molecular degeneration, and need to be moved out of the brain for its healthy function. Vitamin E containing wheat germ mixed with fruits and vegetables, nuts, whole grains, yogurt, in varied combinations can help flush the waste out of the brain. Brain cells need nourishment on daily basis, and this feeding is crucial for the brain to function adequately, and to avoid senility prematurely.

About 100,000 brain cells die each day. To slow down the death rate, as well as to maintain the production of new cells each day require protein feeding to the brain. As long as it is possible, we should see that the cells in our body keep on replicating and forming new ones each day. When cells stop replicating, or the replicating process slows down, we notice aging symptoms all over our body, including the slow down of the brain function.

Avoid Genetic health destiny by learning about family history and taking adequate self managed precautions. It can be postponed or completely avoided by learning the health history of your family which should encompass all the females and males in your father's family, and similarly all the males and females in your mother's family. This will provide you with the genetic pattern of health events that may affect you, so that you can make an attempt to avoid unfavorable health incidents. Eventually, genetic pattern of health will determine the health events in your life, no matter how careful you can be with your diet and life style. You can delay such health events in your life, and may escape them entirely if you are lucky. If you are knowledgeable and prepared then you can avoid the outcomes of such genetic health events.

Now, the key advantage of learning the family health history is to be able to recognize the symptoms of such health events before they occur. First hand knowledge of your own health will provide you with the capabilities to recognize earliest symptoms of the family diseases. This is one of the reasons I stress that in every health event, we must take control of our health and manage it from the beginning to the end. You must know each developing stage of even a common cold. Once you become completely familiar with all the stages and symptoms, it will become quite easy to avoid getting a cold altogether. While the word common cold is in the picture, it is important to know that having more than three colds per year is a serious matter for the patients of stroke, heart disease, and COPD. Do whatever you can to avoid colds. If the specific symptoms of family disease are recognized, there exists a high probability that you will be able to avert it completely, or at least postpone it through deliberate efforts.

***Avoid Anorexia Nervosa** which is a major eating disorder, and is life threatening. Anorexia is lack of appetite and inability to eat. Some women get obsessed with the self induced weight loss programs, and end up reaching 15% to 20% below the adequate weight for their height and age. It is believed that such women have overwhelming fear not to ruin their looks and body shape and, therefore, end up adopting a very low ideal diet. Excessive weight loss may cause hormonal disturbance which may eventually stop their monthly periods prematurely. Anorexia Nervosa should never be taken lightly because it can cause osteoporosis, malnutrition, acute depression with suicidal tendencies, and death.

***Avoiding Bulimia Nervosa**, an abnormally high sensation of hunger which leads to excessive compulsive eating, craving for food, and often thinking of food may help you live a normal life. Ironically, women who suffer from this condition want to look beautiful and slim while at the same time crave food and eat excessively without control. Beside obesity, the individuals suffer from lack of self esteem, feeling of guilt, dependent on medicines, etc.

***Avoid excessive use of Chemicals and Antiseptics** in your living and working quarters for instant cleaning and hygiene. Strong chemicals and antiseptic solutions do eradicate a lot of germs, and make the surfaces shine and biologically safe, however, they create a room and breading ground for more potent germs which can withstand the chemicals and antiseptic in use. First, repeated applications of strong solutions provide a clean and germfree space and invite a new type of germ which was not there before. Secondly, the affected germs keep coming back with new strains with build up resistance to your chemicals and antiseptics, which create higher risks for you. Within a short time span, germs start winning the battle against these strong solutions by developing resistance, and challenging your body's immune system. The best is to use common household soap, or very mild chemicals and very limited antiseptics in combination with a lot of rubbing and scrubbing more frequently. Through labor intensive efforts, you will discourage stronger strains of germs to appear, thereby reducing the degree of danger to your body's immune system. Consequently, your health problems will be reduced significantly.

Avoid bacterial infection through the anus by washing it every day with clean water. Even microscopic residues of feces can attract the invading bacteria thereby causing infection. Such infections remain unnoticed for some time, and can be deadly once colonized inside the colon. Colonized foreign bacteria in colon can destroy the colon wall, and are difficult to eradicate. Infections from fecal residues in the anus can easily spread to vagina due to close proximity in tight clothing. Using antiseptics and other medical solutions will kill the beneficial bacteria which protect the body from the harmful invaders from entering the body. Washing your anus after toilet will prove to be much better than curing various deadly health problems later with unsatisfactory results.

Avoid Bacterial Vaginitis which causes vaginal discharge due to vaginal inflammation. Bacterial infection in the vagina causes vaginal inflammation. In most cases, these discharges are of whitish or yellowish color, and has fishy odor. Although the exact cause is unknown, however, the likely one is related to imbalance between good and bad bacteria. The good and beneficial bacteria protect the body from harmful germs. When the harmful bacteria enter the vagina it disturbs the normal balance, resulting in vaginal discharge. Such vaginal discharges repeat over a period of time. Harmful bacteria enter the vagina through sexual intercourse and inappropriate objects inserted in the vagina. Also, douche (jets) and thongs (strings) can transfer germs from anus to vagina. Appropriate precautions and physician consultations should not be delayed because it is a starting point for many deadly diseases.

Avoid strenuous exercise routine because it can raise the testosterone (not exclusive to men) levels in comparison to estrogen hormones in women over time. This means, in technical sense, that they will become less women than before through the increased testosterone hormone production in their body. There are advantages and disadvantages of being female or male. Increased levels of testosterone production will draw women away from being female, and decrease the chances of their getting pregnant. Of course, women who are obliged to be muscular and very strong due to professional requirements will not be able to avoid heavy workouts in the gym or playground.

Avoid stress tests prescribed by your doctor, because they may cause heart attack or stroke. Women don't need these dangerous tests to find out if they are completely fit. These stress tests put an uneven and enormous stress on body's cardiovascular system in a very short time, which can prove to be extremely dangerous either immediately or within a few days or weeks. You do not want to experience a heart attack or stroke just to find out if you are healthy and fit. Say "no" to stress tests when they are recommended to you. Even if it is determined that you have clogged arteries and require 'bypass surgery' during your regular check ups, stop right there and postpone all decisions until much later. Surgery should be the last option when all other have been examined. One very viable and relatively inexpensive option is Sonogram which is available through several independent sources at about $125, and will provide you with more than adequate data on the arterial blockages, presence of aneurysm, bone-mass evaluation, and the health of your heart. Instantly you will know which precautionary health measures need to be taken.

Even after experiencing a mild heart attack or a mini stroke, you may not require 'bypass surgery'. There are several other alternatives to bypass surgery, which are not difficult to seek. Besides, almost all people have a degree of clogging in their arteries and they have learned and adjusted to live with the condition. Additionally, bypass surgery is good for a few years only and because the arteries will get clogged again and the patient will go for the surgery once again and then again. The best is to take precautions and maintain your wellbeing, seek alternatives to surgery, and if and only if your survival depends upon a surgical procedure then go for it. There is never a guarantee if the surgical procedure will make you healthy, or prolong your life, or you will live through it, or you will ever be in a better health again.

Avoid invasive testing procedures or minimize them. Each invasive testing, like colonoscopy, can expose the innards of the body to air containing all sorts of harmful bacteria. Through invasive testing, the inside of the body may get oxidized giving way to serious health problems that did not exist before. Also, invasive testing can disturb the harmonious chemical and bacterial balance of the body. In other words, any intrusion can disturb the internal environment or the flora and fauna of the body. Proper medical precautions do provide all safeguards against any inadvertent oxidation of some scar, wound, or an ulcer inside the body; but there is no guarantee. Besides, inserting tubes and other devices, it may cause some damage to the inside lining of the organs, which is inherently very soft, delicate, and sensitive.

Some times a noble and necessary medical procedure can bring unexpected and unintended negative outcomes. Always seek an alternative option to invasive testing procedures.

****Avoid unnecessary and futile surgeries*** through prudent decision making which should be based upon thorough research, opinions, degree of necessity, degree of risk, real benefits, recovery time, lifestyle alterations after the surgery, probability of success and, if life-threatening, the survival probability and/ or the extended lifespan, etc. A clear assessment should be made regarding the chances of survival, recuperation, and wellbeing with the surgery verses without the surgery. Several of my healthy and very fit friends died within one year of the surgical procedure, after spending horrible time of recuperation. All of them were diagnosed with some cancer in their body and surgery was strongly recommended to save their lives. The fear of death and hope for long life motivated them to accept the surgical procedures. Often, heart by-pass surgery is recommended to healthy women whose arteries are partially or significantly blocked, but they are not dying or near death. The clogged arteries do pose a serious threat of a stroke or heart attack, but without a life or death emergency leading to the surgical table. Women after the heart by-pass surgery take a long time to recuperate, and are never the same person. Same commentary can be made in other cases of deadly diseases for which the only recommended options happens to be surgery. Besides, after the surgery they are always under the medical discipline with reduced activities, altered lifestyle, and a lot of costly medication.

Surgeries do not provide guarantees that disease wouldn't appear again or no subsequent surgery will be needed or no other disease would replace the previous one. The most practical way for women is to visit a medical facility in a conscious state and voluntarily, and not being hauled away by an ambulance in a panic or semi-conscious state when the medical community gains all the discretions to perform any surgical procedure, necessary or not. Study the survival data, healing data, and body functionality of each surgical procedure much before the chosen surgery to determine if

1) You are seeking exactly what the surgery will accomplish,
2) If it will significantly prolong your life,
3) If the disability and restricted lifestyle acquired after the surgery is acceptable,
4) The chances of your surviving, if you decline the surgical choice over alternative health measures,
5) If you decide to do nothing and continue living your life in the current state of health, and let the chips fall where they may.
6) If you will accept the limited life, prescribed diet, limited mobility, several prescription drugs, future hospital stay and medical visits, future essential or corrective surgeries, associated financial burden, and dependency on others.

MAKE PRUDENT CHOICES

ALCOHOL

Do you know that a moderate amount of ***alcohol***, preferably in the form of red wine, is good for the body? Some researchers believe that any kind of alcohol is good for the body as long the consumption is not more than 2 drinks per day. Alcohol reduces the risk of stroke and heart attacks, it reduces blood clotting. Some alcoholic drinks contain antioxidants like ***catechins*** and ***quercetin*** which help reduce the oxidation of LDL and HDL cholesterols in the body. It increases the levels of good cholesterol (HDL) in the body, if taken in moderation. However, excessive use of alcohol can be bad for stomach lining, liver, and could inhibit omega-3 fatty acids absorption. For most purposes, red and white wines are both beneficial especially to stroke and heart patients. The red grapes with which the red wine is made of contains a unique antioxidant known as ***resveratrol***. Resveratrol is the most effective antioxidant to reduce oxidation of LDL cholesterol in the body, and is found in the skin of red grapes, peanuts, and pistachio nuts.

TEA

There is one drink that has gained acceptability from almost all nutritionists, and that is TEA. Every now and then nutritionists rediscover the good foods and drinks that have been adopted for thousands of years by old cultures. Tea, green or black, is good for you, because it contains several ***antioxidants***. It has been advised that the best way to benefit from drinking tea is without sugar or milk mixed in it. However, there are benefits to be received even if you decide to mix in sugar and milk in your tea. There are two antioxidants that are very special in reducing the risk of stroke and heart attack. These antioxidants are: ***Quercetin***, and ***Catechins.*** Also, tea is very good for the bladder, because it flushing out the viruses and bacteria from the bladder.

CHOCOLATE

There is another great source of ***antioxidants*** and that is chocolate / cocoa. Chocolate is rich in antioxidants, vitamins A & B, iron, calcium, potassium, phosphorus, copper, Chocolate contains ***Phenythelamine*** which is a great stimulant for the brain. Phenythelamine is the ingredient in chocolate that provides the sense of pleasure to the brain. Besides its pleasure giving attributes, it reduces the oxidation of LDL cholesterol. However, consumed in excess may prove to be less beneficial, but rather harmful.

BENEFITING FROM PHYTOCHEMICALS

There are some chemicals in various plant foods, which provide color, aroma and unique fragrance to them. These chemicals are known as Phytochemicals, and they are biologically active. ***Phytochemicals*** do not have any nutritional value, but they do provide resistance against disease to plants. These chemicals are fat free and do not contain any calories, and the medical community does not consider them to be 'essentials'. However, they are some members of the medical community who do think that Phytochemicals could save our lives. Phytochemicals can help prevent and treat a variety of diseases like Cardio Vascular Disease, cancer, menopause, PMS, osteoporosis, prostate problems, and many more. Then there are other parts of plants which are labeled as ***phytonutrients*** which are biologically active, and are 'essentials' for sustaining life.

Free radicals are singular molecules, which roam around in the body to pair up with other molecules. They are ionized, and attract a single electron from a normal cell and destabilize the latter. Quite often, these free radicals attack the cells to pair up with their molecules, and this act can result in disease of some kind. ***Phytochemicals*** that act like ***antioxidants*** save the cells from such attacks by rushing to the site of attack and offering themselves to get paired up. This is a kind of sacrifice to save the cells. A large number of antioxidants in the body will prevent free radicals to attack body cells successfully. However, if antioxidants are in insufficient numbers, free radicals would be able to attack the cells successfully, resulting in decaying of cells and premature aging.

Oxidation occurs when oxygen molecules come in contact with other substances, including body tissue. A cut apple develops a rusty color because molecules of oxygen in the air interact with its molecules. This is similar to a piece of metal which rusts without paint or some other protective coating. The molecules of the cells in the body experience exactly the same chemical interchange when they get exposed to the oxygen containing air and foreign elements. When consumed, the ***antioxidants*** in the fruits and vegetables protect the body cells from getting oxidized.

There are thousands of phytochemicals and many of them are known to science. They serve the body in number of ways. Some of them are: ***Carotenids*** (family of over 450 phytochemicals), is found in leafy vegetables, red and orange fruits. ***Isoflavones*** are found mostly in beans and tofu. ***Isoprenoids*** are mostly found in citrus fruits, carrots, cherries, and whole grains. **Monoterpenes** are found in citrus fruits, cherries, caraway, dill, and spearmint. ***Phytosterols*** are found mostly in peanuts, seeds, and some other nuts. ***Protease Inhibitors*** are found in chick peas, kidney beans, Brussels sprout, broccoli, spinach, corn, seeds, whole grains, potatoes, etc. All vegetables, fruits, nuts, seeds, and herbs contain some type of phytochemical/s, which brings us to the fact established thousands of years ago that in order to stay healthy and prevent disease, one must eat vegetables and fruits of all colors and range, accompanied by all kinds of beans, seeds, nuts, and herbs.

Clinically proven health food intake will not prove to be practical, nor feasible. There are so many nutritional values we want and the sources are numerous, yet we should be able to enjoy the food we eat. Before we can enjoy the food, we have to like it. Each of us have individual taste, metabolism, family history, life style, work habits, physical activity range, financial and social scenario, environment, stress levels, etc. therefore, we should find our own individual functional choices. Once we familiarize ourselves with what is good for us then we will end up making choices which can turn in to habits a little later. The reinforcement of good things in our food choices will definitely make a great difference. In between, we are bound to stray once in a while, and that is alright.

None vegetarians should develop, if already not, a taste and liking for foods which are prepared in combination of several vegetables, beans, grains, fruits, and herbs. There are almost limitless options to suit individual taste buds. You should be able to make your own recipes according your own taste, availability of types of foods, and budget. Visit various eating places, and start looking at different preparations in the light of healthy diet. You will come up with several recipes that you would like to try at home. Learn to enjoy preparing your own favorite meals, no matter how simple they might be. It will be a source of concentration, occupation, creativity, continuous improvisation, skill, and joy. This can turn out to be a great hobby which will feed your body for many decades to come.

Prevent cardio vascular disease by incorporating phytochemicals in your daily diet. It is impossible to eat all the good things that nature provides us to consume to stay healthy, however, we can key phytochemical rich foods in our daily diets. Foods rich in monounsaturated fatty acids, ***soluble fiber*** which is found in oats and beans; ***allicin*** which is found in garlic, folic acid, ***vitamin B6 and vitamin B3*** found in certain fish, bananas, baked potatoes, soy beans, oranges, sunflower seeds, and flaxseeds; ***pectin*** which is found in apples, lentils, spinach, broccoli, brewer's yeast, broccoli, oranges; ***flavonoids*** is found in purple grape juice, ***eritadenine*** is found in shiitake mushrooms.

Capsaicin, found in the hot peppers, protects DNA from carcinogens (cancer causing elements).***Polyphenols***, found in grains, broccoli, parsley, tea, coffee, olive oil, apples, cantaloupe, and most berries; provides protection against free radicals and metals. ***Dindolylmethane***, found in the cabbage family of vegetables, protects the body from many types of cancers. ***Saronins*** is contained in beans and prevents replication of cancer cells in the body. ***Indols*** and ***terpenes***, found in the cabbage family of vegetables, stimulates the production of enzymes that reduce the effectiveness of estrogen in breast cancer risks. There are many other ***phytochemicals*** that provide our body with the protective support against oxidation. Everything that grows in this world has some benefit for our body.

IMPROVING YOUR GENES

The nucleic acids in our body cells are not merely important for the functioning of the body, but are functionally active in determining our biology, characteristics of cells, functional path of cells' health, aging, and just about everything we do and probably what we will do including emotions and behavior. I strongly believe that even the dreams we dream have significant components of the events experienced by our ancestors thousands of years ago. Therefore, it is safe to conclude that no experience or event goes unregistered in our genetic code which is continuously improvising itself at all times ceaselessly in relation to the environment we happen to live in.

Heredity is the program in our DNA, which is continuously changing for the future outcomes. So we have to live by the code that already exists in our DNA and with the code which is being improvised or modified currently, in DNA's future. Our heredity is written in the genetic code whose purpose seems to be to store the procedures or recipe for making protein, because protein carries out just about every chemical, structural, and regulatory function in our body, like digesting food, producing energy, fighting infections, repairing cuts and bruises, etc.

Genetic code can be improved and almost all inherited diseases can be postponed if not entirely avoided by eating, living, behaving, and thinking in the right and most balanced manner. What we eat, think, and do today will be recorded in our genetic makeup, and may be experienced by us in later life, but definitely by the future generations till eternity.

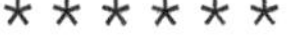

APPENDIX 1

SIGN POSTS OF INFLAMMATION

Our body regenerates the gastro-intestinal lining every 7 to 8 days. This is the natural rhythm of gastro-intestinal system. It is supported by a fatty acid known as '***n-Butyrate***' which provides energy to the cells in the intestinal lining. Low levels indicate that the intestinal lining is under nourished and weak. Weakness in the gastro-intestinal lining points to inflammation and higher risk of colon cancer. Therefore, the intestinal wall should be well nourished with fatty acids through a regular balanced diet.

RISK FACTORS

*Only through the lab tests, the presence of harmful bacteria, if any, in the digestive system is identified. Often, the presence of harmful bacteria is confirmed by the associated enzymes and toxicity which are harmful to the digestive system. An enzyme known as '***beta glucuronidase***' is produced by harmful bacteria, which also indicates that there is high toxicity in the gastro-intestinal tract. According to Dr. John

Furlong, high toxicity and beta-glucuronidase (enzyme) are found in the colon cancer environment.

*Low levels of '***elastase***' indicate insufficient production of ***pancreatic enzymes*** which directly affects the digestion of proteins, fats, sugars, and starches. Low pancreatic enzymes results in incomplete digestion which causes, bloating, weight loss, gas, and even arthritis.

****Calprotectin*** is released by the white blood cells. In the stool tests, if the presence of abnormally high levels of calprotectin is detected then it is the sign of colon cancer, or Crohn's disease, colitis, allergies, polyps, high inflammation, or other related dangers.
*The presence of ***eosinophil protein*** **X** (EPX) indicates that there are parasites in the intestinal tract. Parasites rob the host body of valuable nutrition, and create high toxin levels through its feces in the gut, and resulting in inflammation.

****Sugar***: increased intake of sugar drops the levels of the white blood cells which temporarily suppress body's immune system. Sugar is the favorite food for the increased growth of yeast, bad bacteria, and parasites. High level of sugar intake depletes pancreas and causes insulin burnout, which leads to diabetes. Also, hypoglycemia is linked to excessive consumption of sugar, which results in fatigue, depression, mood changes, etc. Certain yeast and bacteria ferment sugar, and their toxic byproducts end up in the blood stream.

****Nicotine*** causes cancers of lung and the digestive tract. Studies conducted by the *International Agency for Research on Cancer*, France and some researchers in Finland concluded that nicotine smokers of 50 years and over double their risk of getting Colorectal Cancer. Nicotine is an irritant and inflammatory to the intestinal lining, and it weakens the muscles of gastro-esophageal sphincter (the point where esophagus connects to the stomach) due to the reduced production of saliva. Stomach function is impaired due to the decreased blood flow caused by nicotine smoking. Less responsiveness to medicines, and slows down the healing process of intestinal ulcers. The population of free radicals increases in the body, which causes inflammation, infections, gastritis, and ulcers.

****Alcohol*** consumption causes a variety of gastro-intestinal problems including varicose veins in the esophagus, called esophageal varices; gastritis, ulcers, inflammation throughout the digestive tract, liver damage, cirrhosis, compromising pancreas' insulin production ability, etc. Women who consume alcohol habitually run a great risk of numerous health problems.

***Caffeine** which is found in coffee and cocoa is a confirmed irritant, which causes stomach ulcers. It changes the chemistry of the body, and many functions performed by the liver. Caffeine is decidedly an intensifier of the effects produced by the consumption of alcohol, smoking, medication, etc. It can cause cancer of the bladder and pancreas. It is acidic and through stimulation, it increases the acidic level of the stomach. Coffee and cocoa consumption cause loss of valuable minerals like: calcium, magnesium, potassium which are alkaline. Losing these much needed minerals, the body becomes acidic and more prone to inflammation.

***Chemicals and drugs** are another big source of inflammation in the body. These chemicals and drugs which are broadly described as food additives, pesticides, herbicides, preservatives, artificial sugars, etc. They are irritants, inflammatory, and carcinogens. There are thousands of drugs and chemicals we take directly and indirectly, which cause a high level of toxicity in our body and, eventually, the liver ends up with the burden of detoxification process. If the body is overloaded with toxins, the liver will not be able to process them and get rid of them. The toxins which remain in the body get accumulated and cause gastro-intestinal problems like leaky gut, inflammation, cancer, etc.

RECOMMENDATIONS

*Minimizing the intake of canned foods, sugars, hydrogenated fats, processed foods, caffeine, fried foods, dairy products, alcohol, tobacco smoking, junk foods, fast foods, etc is just the first step to restoring health.

*Plenty of water, whole grains, fruits, vegetables, legumes, lentils, nuts, seeds, fermented foods, herbs, cultured foods, eggs, and lean meats should be incorporated in your daily food intakes.

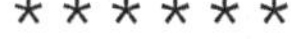

APPENDIX 2

HEALTH PRECAUTIONS WHILE TRAVELING OVERSEAS

It is advisable to take necessary precautions before embarking on a trip overseas. Planning for all eventualities while overseas will provide you with awareness of the conditions prevailing there. The following table will show you the deadliest diseases that are prevalent out in the world, and the toll they inflict upon the population each year. You would not want to catch some disease while traveling overseas, and bring it back home to live with it. The following worldwide figures have been developed by *The World Health Organization.*

Lower respiratory infections (Lungs, bronchial tubes, pneumonia)	4 million die yearly
HIV/AIDS (infection with HIV)	3 million die of AIDS and 39.4 million Live with HIV
Malaria (through mosquitoes)	1 to 5 million die yearly 300 million get affected

Disease	Impact
Diarrhea (bacterial, viral, and parasitic organisms)	2.2 million die, and 2 billion are affected
Tuberculosis (spreads through coughing and sneezing)	2 million die, and 2 billion are infected
Measles (spreads through coughing and sneezing)	530,000 die, and 30 million infected
Whooping cough (highly contagious) (spreads through talking, sneezing and coughing)	200 to 300,000 die, and 20 to 40 million cases
Tetanus (wound infection with bacteria) (attacks central nervous system)	214,000 die, and 500,000 cases
Meningitis (infection of brain and spinal chord tissues) (droplets of throat and breath, close contact)	174,000 die, and 1 million plus cases
Syphilis (a sexual disease through sexual contact)	157,000 die, and 12.2 million Cases

There are several other deadly diseases that are quite common overseas but not in North America, and the travelers may wish to acquaint themselves with various details surrounding them. It is strongly recommended that complete health hazards related information should be obtained from the State Department, travel agencies, and the airlines prior to your departure. Make sure that all the necessary shots have been taken, and all the necessary emergency medication is in your travel bags.

* * * * * *

APPENDIX 3

YEAST INFECTION

There are many kinds of yeast, most of them live peacefully with humans, and however, some, for some strange reasons, become foes and cause ***yeast infection*** or ***candidiasis.*** Candida is a kind of yeast which has a single cell form. The word Candida comes from Latin, meaning "glowing white" because its color is white. There are approximately 600 strains of Candida, and only 25 are known to affect humans.

Candida is everywhere on this planet, and it covers almost everything living. It cohabits with humans and under normal and balanced healthy environment it causes no problems whatsoever. It lives in people under normal and healthy conditions. Under a variety of circumstances, it can grow and get out of control inside the body causing various health problems and disorders like: ***Enteric Candidiasis, Chronic Candida Albicans, Yeast Syndrome, and Candida Related Complex (CRC)*** are just a few.

Normally this yeast is in a round shape, however, when it changes its shape to an oblong one, like hotdog, it is called ***Mycelia***. Mycelia with its oblong shape can dig and embed itself in to the tissue and colonize. This condition is called ***Yeast Infection***, or ***Candidiasis.*** Yeast can penetrate the intestinal lining where it can grow and cause inflammation, through its byproducts (poop). Toxins can weaken the immune system.

Once the immune system is weakened, foreign substances, known as ***Antigens***, can enter the body and weaken it even further. About 79 types of Antigens have been identified and known to enter the body just as soon as the immune system is weakened by Candidiasis or Yeast Infection. Muscle aches, fatigue, headache, fungal infection of the skin and nails, vaginal discharge, infection of urinary canal, premenstrual syndrome, painful breasts, and yeast infection of vagina are some of the common outcomes in women. This is very different from what happens to men when their immune system is weakened through Antigens. Men experience the inflammation of the prostate, benign enlargement of the prostate, loss of libido, agitation, depression, learning disabilities, multiple sclerosis, lupus, psoriasis, and schizophrenia.

CAUSES & RISK FACTORS

There are several known causes for the weakened immune system, and more are expected to be known as research progresses. Some of the causes are listed below:

> *Existence of yeast in the body is normal and remains normal if the body's immune system remains healthy. If the yeast population gets out of control and it starts penetrating the intestinal lining, and infecting and intoxicating the body, then this friendly cohabitant becomes an enemy. Constantly fighting the enemy and having the liver remove growing toxicity on an ongoing basis weakens the immune system.

*Foods and the environment you live in can disrupt this ancient friendship between humans and the yeast. Repeated use of antibiotics to fight infections can lower the immune system. Only specific types of antibiotics can kill specific types of bacteria. When the right antibiotics are used, the targeted bacteria is either killed or stopped from reproducing. Thereafter the use of antibiotics should be stopped for as long as possible, or until the next infection. If the same infection is experienced then it may be somewhat resistant to antibiotics, or may be of different strain for which a new kind of antibiotic may be needed to kill it.

Additionally, antibiotics only target infections, and not the fungi. Bacteria and fungi live in our body in a kind of balance which is disturbed when antibiotics are used or over used, by lowering the population of bacteria. At this time of imbalance, the fungal infection is experienced, and the yeast infection, diarrhea, and gastro-intestinal problems appear. Bacteria keep the fungi at bay, under balanced conditions, and just as soon as antibiotics are used fungal growth increases.

*Packaged white sugars, Confectionery sugars, refined carbohydrates, fruit juices, etc provide an environment for the yeast infection or Candida. Birth control pills, hormonal imbalances from repeated pregnancies, can disrupt the sugar levels in the women's body.

*Also, women on hormone replacement therapy and women with high estrogen levels have high risk levels of having yeast infection.

*Women who smoke or are exposed to tobacco smoke, use medications for ulcers, and are experiencing high stress levels can experience Candida. Appearance of Candida signals intestinal infection and/or presence of intestinal parasites and, therefore, should be tested to alleviate the burden.

*Women whose immune system has already been weakened due to the radiation or chemotherapy for cancer treatment are likely candidates for the yeast infection. Carriers of AIDS virus have a very weak immune system due to various medications and, therefore, are very likely to get yeast infection.

RECOMMENDATIONS

*Live a natural, orderly, and healthy life.
*Take medication only when it is absolutely necessary.
*Avoid taking antibiotics, if possible.
*Stop smoking tobacco and consuming alcohol.
*Learn to depend upon precautions, alternative medications and therapies.
*Maintain personal hygiene.
*Make sure that your dwelling, pantry, air conditioning system, and the appliances are free of fungi, mold, etc.
*Improve your lifestyle, which will improve your immune system.

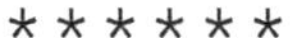

APPENDIX 4

METALS IN YOUR BODY

Metals and toxins can be extremely hazardous to any patient and completely healthy people as well. Metals and toxins tend to clog the blood vessels in one way or another. More importantly, especially metals damage the arterial walls, causing ruptures, inflammation and blood clotting, and blocking or minimizing the flow of blood to the brain. Here is a brief description of each metal which is not only hazardous to the brain but other parts of the body as well.

ALUMINUM

We get Aluminum in our bodies from the cookware, baking powder, aluminum foil, salad dressings, pickles, some ready to serve grated parmesan cheese, some table salts, anti-acids, antiperspirants, various feminine hygiene products, buffered aspirin, canned acidic foods, food additives, lipstick, drugs, medications, processed cheese, softened water, and tap water.

Aluminum targets bones, brains, kidneys, and stomach. Kidney damage, liver dysfunction, loss of appetite, loss of balance, muscle pain, shortness of breath and weakness may signal excess of aluminum in the body. Aluminum causes, neurological disorders like: Alzheimer's disease, Parkinson's disease, senile and pre-senile dementia, staggering while walking, inability to pronounce words properly, memory loss, difficulties in behavior among children in school, etc. Aluminum gets in to the water through acid rain.

Industrial smoke stacks cause release of sulfur in to the atmosphere, which falls back to earth's surface in the form of sulfuric acid. Sulfuric acid kills fish, vegetable life, and threatens humans. Sulfuric acid reacts with various substances in the soil, and turns them in to aluminum, mercury, and lead which get in to the water which we drink. It seems that we are surrounded by aluminum. It is probable that some parts of our brains get destroyed by traces of aluminum which gets in to our bodies from various sources.

Kidney failures may be caused due to the continuous exposure to aluminum, and could warrant use of kidney dialysis regularly. The work of removing waste from the body is taken over by the kidney dialysis from the kidneys. Dialysis involves rinsing out the space between intestines and the intestinal walls with several gallons of fluid, at least, a couple of times a week to remove body waste which would have been carried out by urine in functioning kidneys.

Aluminum can get accumulated in the bone marrow cells responsible for the formation of red blood cells. Consequently, these bone marrow cells are unable to utilize iron, which results in iron deficiency and the negative outcome associated with it. Aluminum can slowly accumulate in our tissues over a life time to cause thinning of bones and brain damage.

ARSENIC

Arsenic is another hazardous substance that is absorbed by our bodies through air pollution, antibiotics given to the commercial live stocks, certain marine plants, chemical processing plants, coal fired power plants, defoliants, drinking water, fish, herbicides, insecticides, meats from commercially raised cattle, poultry, metal ore smelting, pesticides, oysters, mussels, wood preservatives, etc.

Its overall hazardous affect is on all organs, the gastrointestinal system, lungs, skin, etc. Excessive levels of arsenic can cause stomach pain, burning mouth and throat, lung and skin cancer, diarrhea, nausea, skin lesions, peripheral vascular problems, vascular collapse, etc.

CADMIUM

Cadmium comes in to our bodies through the air pollution, art supplies, bone meal, cigarette smoke, coffee, fruit, grains, vegetables grown in cadmium laden soil, highway dust, fungicides, fresh water fish, animal kidneys and livers, refined foods, poultry, incinerators, nickel cadmium batteries, mining, fumes from welding, tobacco and its smoke, sewage sludge, smelting plants, softened water, power plants, phosphate fertilizers, paints, oxide dusts, crabs, flounder, scallops, mussels, oysters, etc.

It adversely affects the brain in general, the pain centers in brain, heart and blood vessels, kidneys and lungs, appetite, etc. It causes anemia, dry and scaly skin, yellow teeth, pain in the back, lung cancer, leg pain, cardio vascular disease, emphysema, fatigue, hair loss, heart disease, joint pain, hypertension, depressed immune system response, kidney stones, liver damage, loss of appetite and sense of smell, etc. Women with any medical history should be especially careful in their diet intakes.

LEAD

We receive lead in our bodies from the air pollution, ammunition (bullets) cast iron porcelain steel bathtubs, canned foods, batteries, chemical fertilizers, ceramics, gasoline, dolomite dust, foods grown around industrial area, cosmetics, hair dyes and rinses, newsprints and color advertisements, leaded glass, paints, pesticides, pewter pottery, rubber toys, soft coal, tobacco smoke, tap water, vinyl mini blinds, etc.

It adversely affects the brain, heart, bones, kidneys, pancreas, liver, nervous system, etc. Lead causes anemia, anorexia, anxiety, stomach pain, exhaustion, brain damage, bone pain, constipation, confusion, dizziness, convulsions, drowsiness, headache, brain damage, hypertension, concentration difficulties, indigestion, loss of appetite, loss of muscle coordination, memory difficulties, miscarriages, etc.

Toxicity of lead is widely known, and even a short time exposure to children and the pregnant women can be dangerous to their health. Still many people believe that once the lead containing paint was banned from their homes, the dangers from lead poisoning were over. Later when lead was banned in gasoline, people thought the danger from lead was completely over. No, it is not over. Lead is in our environment, and people of all income levels, ethnicities, and locations are being affected. This is a great burden on the patients who are trying to get well. Lead is a known neurotoxin which kills brain cells. Higher levels of lead in blood can cause learning disabilities. It causes attention deficit disorder, and reduced intelligence.

MERCURY

Mercury is a known poison. In high or pure doses it is lethal. We receive this poison through the air pollution, batteries, cosmetics, dental amalgams diuretics, electrical devices, relays, explosives, fungicides, grains, fluorescent lights, large bass, pike, trout, large halibut, snappers, sword fish, shrimp, shell fish, tap water, insecticides, pesticides, paints, petroleum products, etc.

Mercury affects the pain centers in the brain, cell membranes, nervous system, kidneys, etc. In excessive levels, Mercury causes abnormality in nervous development, anorexia, anemia, anxiety, blindness, blue line on gums, depression, colitis, dermatitis, difficulty in chewing and swallowing, depression, dizziness, drowsiness, hypertension, headache, emotional instability, nerve damage, memory loss, vision impairment, inflamed gums, insomnia, kidney damage, metallic taste, loss of smell, hearing loss, hallucinations, fatigue, fever, loss of appetite, loss of muscles, loss of weight, etc.

Among the main sources of exposure to Mercury is from the silver dental fillings. Fillings contain about 50% mercury when placed in teeth. Mercury fillings release microscopic particles and vapors of mercury each and every time a person chews. Particles get absorbed and the vapors are inhaled. Mercury particles absorption takes place in tooth roots, mucous membranes of the mouth and gums, and in the stomach lining. Mercury levels range between 20 and 400 mcg/m3 in the mouth and there remains a continuous exposure.

Various researches have been conducted on the affects of mercury in the dental fillings, with varied outcomes. A common outcome has been the experience of depression, suicidal impulses, irritability, inability to cope, muscle spasms, seizures, multiple sclerosis, cardio vascular problems, accelerated heart beat, facial tics, arthritis, bursitis, immune system diseases, airborne allergies, food allergies, effects on psychological reactions, etc.

NICKEL

Yet there is another metal which is hazardous. It is Nickel. You receive exposure to nickel from the cooking utensils, ceramics, appliances, cocoa, coins, cosmetics, dental materials, hydrogenated oils, chocolate, nuts, foods grown near industrial areas, industrial waste, hair spray, medical implants, jewelry, metal refineries, nickel cadmium batteries, metal tools, orthodontic appliances, shampoos, solid waste incinerators, kitchen utensils made of stainless steel, tap water, tobacco and its smoke, water faucets and pipes, zippers, etc.

Nickel affects the larynx (voice box), the areas of skin exposed to it, lungs, nasal passages, etc. Nickel causes blue colored lips, shortness of breath, vomiting, headache, rapid heart rate, shortness of breath, skin rashes, insomnia, diarrhea, fever, cancer of lung, larynx and nasal passage, gingivitis, etc. This proves that it is not an easy task to get well fast when a woman patient has to face so many dangers from so many sources at once, besides the health danger from within. It is the accumulative burden that is so burdensome on any woman, making it a compelling reason for her to be as cautious as the circumstances allow.

RECOMMENDATIONS

Over the years, people have known that clean blood means good health. Chemicals, toxins, excessive fat, calcium, plaque, excessive minerals and metals, etc. block the flow of blood. The Chelation therapy has been suggested to reduce calcium and plaque lodged on the arterial walls. The atherosclerotic plaque can occur in any artery of the body, and is not limited to the arteries near the brain or heart. This plaque can stop or reduce the flow of blood. Blood carries oxygen to various parts of the body. The lack of oxygen results in dead cells. There are over 75,000 miles of blood vessels in our body, largest ones to the smallest ones, which supply blood to every cell tissue, gland, and organ in the body.

Organic acids naturally found in our bodies and in foods can act as Chelating agents, including acetic acid, ascorbic acid (vitamin C), citric and lactic acids. Natural chelating process allows us to experience digestion, assimilation and transportation of food nutrients, along with the formation of enzymes, and hormones, and detoxification of toxic chemicals and metals. Nature does it all by itself.

Chelating therapy is inter venous and involves injecting chelating agents in to the blood stream to eliminate undesirable substances like the heavy metal, chemicals, toxins, mineral deposits and fatty plaques. In this therapy process, EDTA (***Ethylene Diamine Tetra acetic Acid***) is injected in the bloodstream. The Chelating agents (EDTA) are substances which can chemically bond with metals, minerals, chemical toxins, etc. In fact these agents encircle the ions of metals, minerals, chemicals, toxins, and carry them out of the body via the urine and feces.

Chelating therapy with EDTA was first introduced in the USA in 1948 as a treatment for Lead Poisoning, Workers were found to have lead poisoning caused by the environment of Battery Factory where they worked. Later, several Naval Sailors were treated for lead poisoning for having subjected to painting the ships and other facilities. Physicians who were treating these workers in the battery factory and naval sailors who were painting ships, with chelating therapy, were surprised that patients who also had Atherosclerosis (fatty plaque built up in the arterial walls) or Arteriosclerosis (hardening of the arteries) experienced reduction in both conditions. The Chelating therapy with EDTA has been reportedly successful with numerous beneficial effects, however, before giving it any consideration, check with your personal physician if it is workable for you.

Some of benefits of Chelating Therapy are:

*Reduction in blood clumping and preventing blood clots, marked improvement in patients with vascular diseases improved cognitive function in people with memory and concentration deficits, improved visual acuity (specially when problem caused by arterial blockages), reduction of blood fat levels, improved and increased blood flow to extremities of the body, decalcification of elastic tissue resulting in improved elasticity and resilience, decreased blood pressure levels, various levels of benefits for aneurysm, Alzheimer, senile dementia, arthritis, diabetes, osteoporosis, Parkinson disease, varicose veins, stroke, venomous snake bites, etc.

*Amazingly, 90% of Americans face danger from illness related to blood circulatory system. *The American Heart Association* estimates that the treatment of CVD alone costs more than $ 475 Billion annually, and an estimated cost of a bypass surgery is more than $400,000 per case. Inter venous Chelating therapy is far less invasive and expense driven. But there is one danger associated with Chelating therapy which may lower the levels of calcium in the bones and teeth. To replace the calcium drawn from the blood by Chelating therapy with EDTA, body will draw calcium from bones and teeth to replace it. A thorough testing and approval by your personal physician will be required before undertaking such a therapy.

Oral Chelation is when nutritious food supplements in combination with certain chelating agents, like EDTA and other natural chelators, including vitamins, minerals, amino acids, antioxidants, and herbs are taken on a scheduled basis. It is quite affective. In spite of the fact that it is a much slower method but it will accomplish the same as inter venous chelating would. It is believed to reduce heavy metal toxicity and calcification, it will lower cholesterol, it will reduce free radical oxidation of metabolized fats, it will prevent formation of blood clots, etc. Your doctor will be the best to judge if it is a suitable therapy for you.

Some of these nutrients may protect you against heavy metal absorption and toxicity. You may take magnesium to ward off the ill affects of aluminum. To avoid ill affects of arsenic in your body, try taking amino acids with sulfur, calcium, iodine, selenium, vitamin C, and zinc. Cadmium absorption can be minimized by taking amino acids with sulfur, calcium, vitamin C, and zinc. The absorption of lead in the body can be minimized by taking amino acids including sulfur, pectin (alginate), selenium, vitamin C, There are several oral chelating formulas developed by medical professionals over the years, with primarily one objective and that is to remove metals and toxins from the body. You may wish to explore this with your doctor before making any decision in this regard.

Other measures include moving away from the industrial zone, crowded areas, and the big cities, and living and working in a very small town environment. In other words, going back to nature and living a very simple life without the luxuries and comforts of modern lifestyle, shopping malls, manufactured foods, jobs with good salaries, cars, buses, commuter trains, workshops, etc may be an alternative, but may not be workable for most women.

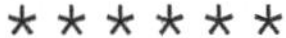

APPENDIX 5

DENTAL TOXICITY

Most people in the United States have had some dental work done on their teeth requiring some sealants, amalgams, composites, etc. Dental fillings contain mercury and several other toxic substances when placed in teeth, which release microscopic particles and vapors. The effect of these procedures can be experienced throughout the body in major organs, which may cause a variety of associated illnesses such as fatigue, difficulty in concentration, allergies, depression, asthma, arthritis, skin disorders, etc.

Toxins from dental amalgams, cements, composites, varnishes, sealants, pastes, adhesives, etc. can cause Heavy Metal Toxicity. Sealants cause ***Neurocutaneous Syndrome*** (NCS) which degrades the skin and the neurological system of the patients who have been treated with sealants during filling or root canal procedures, says Dr. Omar Amin of Arizona. Brain fog and loss of memory may be experienced by patients. Small itchy sores or inflamed pimples with tendency to spread may appear. General symptoms include compromised immune system, fatigue, and psychological trauma.

* * * * * *

APPENDIX 6

MEDICAL ERRORS

On a daily basis medical errors are committed in diagnosis, prognosis, tests, prescriptions, etc by medical communities throughout the country in spite of concerted efforts to monitor each step of the patients' treatment at the clinics and medical facilities. Errors are committed by all humans during the performance of daily chores, performing job related duties, etc but most of them are not life threatening. Dealing with patients' health condition and the wellbeing of average person, every error committed by the medical community is life threatening. All should be extra vigilant from the dangers of errors on the part of doctors, nurses, specialists, radiologists, testing labs, and even the staff members performing other duties within the medical facility.

Every year, a huge number of people die or get sick, or become disabled due to errors committed by medical professionals and their staff members. Various estimates have been put forth to determine the incidence of medical mistakes over the course of time, but all have been partial or incomplete. No doubt it is very hard to determine exactly how many patients and healthy people get affected or die, because the proximate causes of death or sickness through medical errors are difficult to define and pinpointed. There are numerous contributory factors that surround such incidents and therefore make assessments somewhat vague and nebulous.

According to *the National Academy of Sciences, Institute of Medicine of the National Academies, medical errors harm many Americans.*

> *At least 1.5 million Americans are harmed by medical errors each year at a conservatively estimated cost of $3.5 billion
> *400,000 preventable drug related injuries occur in the hospitals, each year
> *800,000 preventable injuries occur in long term care setting, each year
> *530,000 injuries occur among Medicare recipients in out patient clinics, each year

These Institutes of the National Academies admitted that these are most likely to be under estimates of the exact incidence of mistakes.

Health Grade Studies of Colorado claims that medical errors cost $8.8 billion, and result in 238,337 preventable deaths each year. WrongDiagnosis.com claims that about 225,000 die due to medical errors, each year in the U.S.A.

Barbara Starfield's article in JAMA (*Journal of American Medical Association*), 225,000 deaths occur each year due to iatrogenic causes (resulting from patients' treatment by a physician or surgeon) which would make it 3rd leading cause of death in the U.S.A.

About 2 million cases of various types of infections occur annually among hospital patients, which is about 10% of the total patient population in the hospitals.

42% of the people in the U.S.A believe that they personally experienced medical mistakes

*affecting them personally	33%
*a relative	48%
*a friend	19%

Encyclopedia.com claims that 1 in 5 deaths in the USA is due to misdiagnosis, 195.000 die from medical errors, According to AHRQ (*Agency for Healthcare Research & Quality*, says that medical errors cost USA $37 billion per year. The reasons of all these errors may be linked to the

*lack of adequate qualification and training
*carelessness
*unstable and destructive personality
*lack of ethical values
*dollar based healthcare system where highest revenue generating treatment, surgeries, medications, etc will get promoted rather than the wellbeing of patients

*tiredness on the part of over worked medical staff
*excessive pressure from the corporations controlling the medical community to operate within certain cost parameters to produce higher revenues, thereby negatively effecting the welfare of patients
*profit based healthcare creates an inducement for the medical community to seek ways and methods to intensively cultivate patients for higher revenues

*business models upon which hospitals, clinics, testing laboratories, etc operate on "average patient billing" method, compels them to aspire to increase the average billing amount as soon as it is possible

*under business environment, no doubt the medical community puts emphasis on high revenue producing surgical procedures much more than alternative treatment methods.

*higher legal costs have compelled the medical community to cut costs which may have resulted in lower quality of healthcare at some places

RECOMMENDATIONS

*Wash your hands several times a day, but especially after visiting a medical facility.

*Minimize your visits to your doctor's office, hospital, medical laboratory, etc unless it is absolutely necessary.

*Upon returning home after visiting your doctor or a hospital, take a shower and use soap.

*Make an effort to wash your system with plenty of water and other liquids after visiting a medical facility.

*Contact your doctor over the phone immediately should you find yourself not feeling well.

*Tell your doctor about your allergies, current medications, diet, health condition, etc in detail so that your doctor becomes aware of your health condition completely.

*Question each test you are subjected to take, and avoid unnecessary tests.

*Study each test result you receive from your doctor, and seek explanations.

*Your doctor's advice, prescriptions, precautions, medication method, diet, instructions, etc must be written in legible handwriting which is completely understood by you and, hopefully, by the pharmacist.

*Get advised of the side effects and possible reactions to all the medication prescribed by your doctor, in writing.
*Instead of relinquishing control of your healthcare to your doctor, or nurse, or the pharmacist, you should take control in your own hands and make the doctor and the medical staff help you manage it. It is your body and your life, therefore, you need to control and manage it because you care the most.
*Make sure that you are picking up, or being delivered, the correct medicine prescribed by your doctor.

*During any physical contact with your body, don't hesitate to ask your doctor, nurse, or other medical staff if they washed their hands. They may have handled some other patient with some life threatening infection just before they came to see you.
*Make sure that you, your doctor, specialist, surgeon, nurses, and other medical staff are absolutely sure about your surgical procedure prior to your sedation, because surgeries cannot be undone. Through errors some patients lose their limbs, organs, etc through instructional mix ups and carelessness.

*Obtain a written advice on after-surgery-care at home or elsewhere with dos and don'ts.
*Ask questions repeatedly until you feel satisfied, and if you don't understand something, or feel convinced then don't agree to it. Postpone your decision until you fully understand the issue, procedure, advice, etc.
*Make sure to find out why your doctor and the specialist want you to go through a certain surgery, or remove an organ, or something permanent like that. Take second third and fourth opinions.

*Many surgeries can be avoided because there are always some alternatives which need to be explored and discussed.
*Your doctor should be the overall in-charge of your surgery

even though the surgery is performed by a surgeon after the recommendation of a specialist.

*Make sure that your complete medical history, diagnosis; prognosis, treatment, current medication, allergies, blood tests, etc are available with the surgeon prior to sedation.

*Try your best to have a conscientious and alert family member, or a dear friend present during surgical procedure.

*Leave the hospital or medical clinic immediately, each and every time, you are allowed because you don't want to catch some infection and bring it home.

******

APPENDIX 7

GLANDS & HORMONES

Hormones are chemical substances formed in various glands in the body and are secreted out, which have specific regulatory effects on certain cells, organs, and tissue.

All hormones are essential to the body and there are many that are produced by various organs. The major ones are:

*__*Cortisol hormone*__, secreted by the adrenal gland, helps the body to combat stress, reduces inflammatory response of the body, and mobilizes fats for energy in the body.

*__*Erythropoietin hormone*__, produced by the kidneys, stimulates the production of red blood cells for the bone marrow.

*__*Gastrin hormone*__, secreted by the stomach, stimulates the production of hydrochloric acid to break down food for digestion.

***Growth hormone**, secreted by the pituitary gland, stimulates growth of the liver, muscles, bones, and cartilages in the body

***Insulin,** produced by the pancreas, helps feed glucose to the cells, instrumental in the cell receptors' ability to take glucose from the bloodstream inside the cell membrane, lowers the blood sugar levels

***Leptin hormone**, produced by the adipose tissue, helps control appetite in the brain, regulates the body fat storage, metabolism, and the absorption of sugars.

***Thyroid hormone**, produced by the thyroid gland, regulates the blood pressure, promotes the development and maintenance of the nervous system, muscles, metabolism and the body skeleton; and regulates the moisture in the skin.

Hormones play a key role in replication and production of cells in our body. Hormones build walls and the inner components of the cells. All glands secrete moisture which is mostly protein suitable for the body cells to ingest. This moisture is called hormones which are fed to millions of cells and tissues in our body. This process of hormone feeding to the body cells and tissues creates and promotes replication and regeneration of cells, which is absolutely necessary to offset the cell decay and aging process, at least to some extent.

There are several glands which require regular supply of protein for adequate health and functioning. Hence, protein in our diet becomes essential for the adequate supply of hormones in our body, which in fact promotes the youthfulness in our physical and mental self. Glands and hormones are mostly protein. All glands in our body work in harmony in relation to each other. If one gland is functioning inadequately, then all other glands become sluggish and less than adequate in function. Therefore, harmony among glands is essential. This essential harmony among glands can easily be accomplished by moderate, regular and sustainable physical activity which employs all body functions like household work, gardening, farming, playing a sport, aerobics, etc. There are many glands in our body including more than 2 million sweat glands in the skin; however, the prominent ones that affect our health are as follows:

Thyroid gland, located at the base of the throat in front of the wind pipe, uses protein from our daily diet and, in return, produces ***Thyroxin,*** an important hormone. Thyroxin regulates the consumption of food in our body, usage of oxygen, rate at which our bodies process the food and the metabolism in general. It provides protein nourishment to the body cells and tissues, and moistens the skin to give it a younger appearance. It is a kind of rejuvenating hormone. Lack or insufficient quantities of Thyroxin, can cause a condition called ***hypothyroid*** which could make our brains to slow down, make us look older prematurely, adversely affect the digestive system, tiredness and other related symptoms may appear. To feed your brain and put some gusto in the body, it is recommended that protein be taken in combination with vegetables containing iodine. There are some ocean fish that are high in protein and iodine, but that could be expensive as well as may contain other undesirable substances due to chemical and toxic pollution in the environment. Again, this combination will stimulate the brain, and may help prevent various diseases.

****Pituitary gland,*** located at the base of the brain, also called the master gland, uses protein to produce about 9 hormones to stimulate hypothalamus. One of the hormones produced in this chain process is ***ACTH*** which is known to create a defense mechanism against arthritis. ACTH is also known to stimulate the adrenal gland to produce various hormones like ***hydrocortisone*** which is a natural arthritis defense. Hormones produced by pituitary gland controls, to a great extent, the muscles, skeleton, tendons, etc. Combination of plant protein and animal protein is an adequate way to feed the pituitary gland which produces at least nine hormones which help women to strengthen their tendons, muscles, and the body in general.

Adrenal glands*, located next to the kidneys, produce hormone known as ***adrenalin.* Adrenalin provides a kind of instant alert to the nerves and muscles in the body. It helps build up and sharpen the reflexes. It improves vision, hearing, nerves, heart, muscles, removal of toxins, stress, etc. A combination of protein foods mixed with the vitamin C containing foods is recommended to feed the adrenal glands. ***Cortisol*** hormone, secreted by adrenal gland, helps body to combat stress, reduces inflammatory response of the body, and mobilizes fats for energy in the body.

Pancreas*, located behind the lower section of the stomach, like sweetbread in animals, produces hormone known as Insulin. ***Insulin* helps the blood to convert sugar as it is needed by the body. Insulin, produced by pancreas, helps feed glucose to body cells, instrumental in cell receptors' ability to take glucose from the bloodstream to inside of the cell membrane, and lowers the blood sugar levels in the bloodstream.

Insulin production must be adequate and consistent, so that the exact amount of sugar is provided to the body cells. Consuming too much fat and sugar, and not enough protein, leads the pancreas to overwork which leads to weakness of pancreas, and then it fails to produce adequate amounts of insulin to regulate the blood sugar when needed. When sugar does not get burned and regulated, diabetes sets in. Besides, reducing fats and sugars in the diet, adequate nourishment needs to be provided to the pancreas to continuously produce insulin. A combination of protein from animal and plant source and carbohydrates from plant source is recommended.

Sex glands: female sex glands are the ovaries located in the lower region of women, which makes it possible to reproduce and give birth. Female sex glands produce two hormones: ***estrogen*** and ***progesterone*** which provide women the fertility and the pretty and delicate looks. A combination of animal protein, plant protein, and vegetables is recommended for adequate supply of estrogen and progesterone.

****Parathyroid glands***, total 4 in number, located around the thyroid gland just in front of the wind pipe. Parathyroid glands produce hormone known as ***parathormone*** which helps to regulate the use of phosphorus and calcium in the body. Lack of sufficient ***parathormone*** in the body may produce nervous instability, uncontrollable rage and anger, sudden outbursts, and other emotional irregularities, besides osteoporosis related problems. A combination of foods containing protein, calcium, and phosphorous is recommended.

****Thymus gland,*** located just below thyroid gland at the base of the neck, produces a number of hormones which stimulate the metabolism of minerals, calcium, and phosphorous. Thymus hormones feed the brain with protein, and protect it from senility. Thymus hormones manufacture white blood corpuscles which become a natural guard against infections. These hormones also build and repair red blood cells which aid in the healing process. Most definitely, they improve mental alertness which aging women need. A combination of grains, wheat germ, and fruits is recommended for a healthy thymus.

Sufficient quantities of protein from plant and dairy sources is available in beans, tofu, grains, nuts, cheeses, milk, etc which can be easily incorporated in the daily food intake.

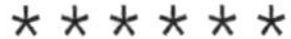

APPENDIX 8

PLATELETS

Blood platelets, known in medical terms as ***thrombocytes*** are absolute essentials for the body's normal blood coagulation. They are tiny fragments of a larger cell in the bone marrow, called ***megakaryocyte***. Platelets provide protective services to the body by patching the damaged or cut areas with a thick patch of coagulated blood. When there is even a very small cut and the blood oozes out, the platelets stop the bleeding by forming a dam of thick and congealed blood, which stops he bleeding. In the absence of such a patchwork, the body will not stop bleeding.

According to Dr. Richard Fogorus, platelets travel the blood stream, and when any bleeding occurs an instant chemical reaction changes the surface of platelets making it sticky and gluey. Once chemically activated they start sticking to the site of bleeding and within a short time a clump of platelets appear on it. The subsequent chemical reaction produces a substance called ***fibrin*** which is stringy web like complex of strands. The red blood cells are caught in the web and a red clot is formed. This blood clot stops the bleeding. However, these blood clots are very dangerous if formed within the arteries and veins, which obstruct the normal blood flow. Another very dangerous situation occurs when they protect an ulcer underneath a plaque, and/or a portion of plaque gets dislodged and debris is resulted in the process of stopping bleeding. When activated platelets encase the plaque debris, the resultant blood clots can cause serious damage to the body including the heart and brain.

Platelets are always present in a healthy or normal bloodstream, and range anywhere from 700,000 to 1,000,000 per cubic millimeter of blood. Women with lower count of platelets will experience frequent bleeding even from a small cut which will take longer to heal.

Women with platelet count as low as 50,000 per cubic millimeter may experience small hemorrhages, bleeding from tiny blood vessels in the skin, large or small purplish patches beneath the skin, black and blue spots on the skin, nose bleeding, bleeding in gums, gastrointestinal hemorrhages, urinary bleeding, and abnormally longer menstruation periods, etc. Women with these symptoms should be extra careful being out because any substantial accident related injury can be life threatening. On the other hand, if the platelets are too high (700,000 or higher) then certain types of cancer, anemia, heart disease, leukemia, and stroke, etc. may occur.

Although personal physician should be contacted to explore the cause of these symptoms, this could be cured by sufficient doses of Vitamin K and Vitamin C. When the platelets remain at low levels, a study of the mother cell ***megakyocyte*** in the bone marrow is conducted by the doctor to determine if it is capable of producing sufficient number of platelets. Such a test is conducted because many industrial chemicals and certain medications may be toxic to the mother cell.

Presence of sufficient numbers of platelets is extremely important for survival, especially during surgical procedures. Excessive or non-stop bleeding can be an exhaustive challenge for the surgeon and a life threatening event for the patient with insufficiency in platelet count.

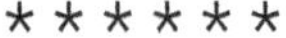

APPENDIX 9

NUTRITIONAL VALUES

Foods you should incorporate in your diet for better health

BEANS & LENTILS

BLACK BEANS (one cup cooked & drained) contains 15 grams of protein, 47 mg of calcium, 239 mg of phosphorus, 2.9 mg of iron, and 609 mg pf potassium

GREAT NORTHER BEANS (one cup cooked & drained): 14 grams of protein, 90 mg of calcium, 266 mg of phosphorus, 4.9 mg of iron, and 749 mg of potassium,

CHICK PEAS (one cup cooked & drained): contains 15 grams of protein, 80 mg of calcium, 273 mg of phosphorus, 4.9 mg of iron, and 475 mg of potassium.

LENTILS: (one cup cooked & drained): contains 16 grams of protein, 50 mg of calcium, 238 mg of phosphorus, 4.2 mg of iron, 498 mg of potassium, 40 IU of vitamin A

SOYBEANS (one cup cooked & drained): contains 20 grams of protein, 131 mg of calcium, 322 mg of phosphorus, 4.9 mg of iron, 972 mg of potassium, 50 IU of vitamin A

Besides very nutritious **Moong Bean, Kidney Beans, Pinto Be**ans, there is a large variety of other beans and lentils in the marketplace.

NUTS & SEEDS

ALMONDS: 1 ounce (about 24 whole almonds) contains 6 grams of protein, 3.35 grams of fiber, 8.2 mcg of foliate, 7.3 mg of vitamin E, 2.8 I.U. of vitamin A, 1.1 mg of niacin, 206 mg of potassium, 134 mg of phosphorus, 70 mg of calcium, 0.2 mg of sodium, 77 mg of magnesium, 1.2 mcg of selenium, 1.2 mg of iron, 0.95 mg of zinc, 0.7 mg of manganese,

BRAZIL NUTS: one ounce (about 7 whole nuts) contains 4 grams of protein, 2.1 grams of fiber, 6.24 mcg of foliate, 1.6 mg of vitamin E, 1.0 mg of vitamin C, 205 mg of phosphorus, 186.8 mg of potassium, 106 mg of magnesium, 543 mcg of selenium, 45 mg of calcium, 1.15 mg of zinc, and 0.69 mg of iron

CASHEW NUTS:: one ounce raw whole nuts contains 5.17 grams of protein, 0.94 gm of fiber, 9.7 mcg of vitamin K, 7.0 mcg of foliate, 187 mg of potassium, 168 mg of phosphorus, 82.8 mg of magnesium, 10.5 mg of calcium, 3.4 mg of sodium, 1.9 mg of iron, and 1.64 mg of zinc, and 5.6 mg of selenium.

CHESTNUTS: 10 roasted kernels with no salt added contain 2.7 grams of protein, 4.3 grams of fiber, 20 I.U. of vitamin A, 21.8 mg of vitamin C, 1.12 mg of niacin, 0.46 mg of pantothenic acid, 58.8 mcg of foliate, 6.55 mcg of vitamin K, 497 mg of potassium, 90 mg of phosphorus, 24.4 mg of calcium, 27.7 mg of magnesium,

1.7 mg of sodium, 0.76 mg of iron, 1.0 mcg of selenium, 1.0 mg of manganese,

HAZELNUTS: 10 raw nuts contain 2 grams of protein, 1.4 grams of fiber, 2.8 I.U. of vitamin A, 0.9 mg of vitamin C, 15.8 mcg of foliate, 2 mcg of vitamin K, 95 mg of potassium, 40.6 mg of phosphorus, 22.8 mg of magnesium, 16 mg of calcium, 0.66 mg of iron.

MACADAMIA NUTS: one ounce (about 11 kernels), raw, contains 2.24 grams of protein, 2.44 grams of fiber, 3.1 mcg of foliate, 104 mg of potassium, 53 mg of phosphorus, 36.9 mg of magnesium, 24 mg of calcium, 1.4 mg of sodium, 1.0 mg of iron.

PECANS: one ounce (about 20 halves), raw, contains 2.6 grams of protein, 2.7 grams of fiber, 15.8 I.U. of vitamin A, 6.23 mcg of foliate, 116 mg of potassium, 78 gm of phosphorus, 34.3 mg of magnesium, 19.8 mg of calcium, 1.3 mg of zinc, 0.7 mg of iron, 1.3 mg of manganese, 1.0 mcg of selenium.

PEANUTS: one ounce raw contains 7.3 grams of protein, 1.0 gm of fiber, 3.4 mg of niacin, 3.4 mg of vitamin E, 68 mcg of foliate, 200 mg of potassium, 107 mg of phosphorus, 47.6 mg of magnesium, 26 mg of calcium, 5.1 mg of sodium, 1.3 mg of iron, 2.0 mcg of selenium.

PINE NUTS: one ounce contains 3.9 grams of protein, 1.0 gram of fiber, 2.6 mg of vitamin E, 1.2 mg of niacin, 19 mcg of foliate, 8.2 I.U. of vitamin A, 15.3 mcg of vitamin K, 169 mg of potassium, 163 mg of phosphorus, 71 mg of magnesium, 4.5 mg of calcium, 2.4 mg of manganese, 1.8 mg of zinc, 1.6 mg of iron.

PISTACIO NUTS: one ounce (about 49 kernels) dry roasted contains 6.0 grams of protein, 3.0 grams of fiber, 74.3 I.U. of vitamin A, 14.2 mcg of foliate, 295.4 mg of potassium, 137 mg of phosphorus, 34 mg of magnesium, 31.2 mg of calcium, 2.8 mg of sodium, 1.2 mg of iron, 2.6 mcg of selenium.

PUMPKIN SEEDS: one ounce roasted without salt contains 5.3 grams of protein, no fiber, 17.6 I.U. of vitamin A, 2.6 mcg of foliate, 260 mg of potassium, 74 gm of magnesium, 26 mg of phosphorus, 15.6 mg of calcium, 5.1 mg of sodium, 2.9 mg of zinc, 0.9 mg of iron.

SUNFLOWER SEEDS: one ounce, dry roasted, contains 5.5 grams of protein, 3.1 mg of fiber, 6.5 I.U. of vitamin A, 67.2 mcg of foliate, 6.0 mg of vitamin E, 327.2 mg of phosphorus, 241 mg of potassium, 36.6 mg of magnesium, 19.8 mg of calcium, 1.5 mg of zinc, 0.9 mg of iron.

WALNUTS: one ounce, (about 14 halves) contains 4.3 grams of protein, 1.9 mg of fiber, 27.8 mcg of foliate, 125 mg of potassium, 98.0 mg of phosphorus, 44.8 mg of magnesium, 27.8 mg of calcium, 1.0 mg of zinc, 0.8 mg of iron, 1.4 mcg of selenium.

FRUITS

APPLE: one medium apple with skin contains no protein, 4 grams of fiber, 73 I.U. of vitamin A, 9 mg of vitamin C, 4 mcg of foliate, 0.66 I.U. of vitamin E, 158 mg of potassium, 9.5 mg of calcium, 9.5 mg of phosphorus, 7 mg of magnesium, and 4 mg of selenium.

AVOCADO: one medium, contains 4 grams of protein, 10 gm of fiber, 1230 I.U. of vitamin A, 15.9 mg of vitamin C, 3.9 mg of niacin, 124 mcg of foliate, 1.9 mg of pentothenic acid, 0.56 mg of vitamin B6, 0.2 mg of vitamin B1, 0.25 mg of vitamin B2, 1204 mg of potassium, 82.4 mg of phosphorus, 78.4 mg of magnesium, 22 mg of calcium, 20 mg of sodium, 2 mg of iron.

BANANA: one medium, contains 1 gram of protein, 3 grams of fiber, 95 I.U. of vitamin A, 11 mg of vitamin C, 22.5 mcg of foliate, 0.7 mg of vitamin B6, 0.6 mg of niacin, 0.31 mcg of pentothenic acid, 0.67 mg of vitamin E, 467 mg of potassium, 43 mg of magnesium, 27 mg of phosphorus, 7 mg of calcium, 1.3 mg of selenium, 0.4 mg of iron.

BLACKBERRIES: one cup contains 1 gram of protein, 7 grams of fiber, 237 I.U. of vitamin A, 30 mg of vitamin C, 1.5 mg of vitamin E, 49 mcg of foliate, 282 mg of potassium, 46 mg of calcium, 30 mg of phosphorus, 28 mg of magnesium, 1.9 mg of manganese, 0.8 mg of iron, 0.9 mg of selenium, 0.4 mg of zinc.

CANTALOUPE: one medium slice contains 0.6 grams of protein, 0.55 grams of fiber, 2225 I.U. of vitamin A, 3.7 mg of vitamin C, 3.9 mg of foliate, 0.4 mg of niacin, 213 mg of potassium, 12 mg of phosphorus, 7.6 mg of calcium, 7.6 mg of magnesium.

GRAPES; one cup contains one gram of protein, 1.6 grams of fiber, 92 I.U. of vitamin A, 3.7 mg of vitamin C, 3.6 mcg of foliate, 176 mg of potassium, 13 mg of calcium, 9 mg of phosphorus, 4.6 mg of magnesium, 0.4 mg of iron, 0.3 mg of selenium.

KIWI: one cup contains 1.75 grams of protein, 6 grams of fiber, 310 I.U. of vitamin A, 174 mg of vitamin C, 67 mcg of foliate, 3 I.U of vitamin E, less than 1 mg of vitamins B2 and B6, 0.9 mg of niacin, 588 mg of potassium, 71 mg of phosphorus, 53 mg of magnesium, 46 mg of calcium, 1.1 mg of selenium, 0.72 mg of iron, 0.3 mg of zinc, 0.3 mg of copper.

LEMON: one without peel contains .64 grams of protein, 1.6 grams of fiber, 2 I.U. of vitamin A, 4 mg of vitamin C, 80 mg of potassium, 15 mg of calcium, 9.2 mg of phosphorus, 4.6 mg of magnesium, 0.35 mg of iron,.

LIME: one, without peel, contains 0.4 grams of protein, 1.8 grams of fiber, 6.7 I.U of vitamin A, 19 mg of vitamin C, 5.5 mcg of foliate, 68 mg of potassium, 22 mg of calcium, 12 mg of phosphorus, 4 mg of magnesium, 0.4 mg of iron.

MANGO; one without the peel, contains 1 gram of protein, 3 grams of fiber, 8060 I.U. of vitamin A, 57 mg of vitamin C, 29 mcg of foliate, 1.2 mg of niacin, 3.51 I.U of vitamin E, less than 1 mg each of vitamins B2 and B6, 323 mg of potassium, 20.7 mg of calcium, 22.8 mg of phosphorus, 18.6 mg of magnesium, 0.26 mg of iron.

ORANGE: one medium, contains 1 gram of protein, 3 grams of fiber, 269 I.U. of vitamin A, 70 mg of vitamin C, 40 mcg of foliate, less than 1 mg each of vitamin B1 and pantothenic acid, 237 mg of potassium, 52 mg of calcium, 18 mg of magnesium, 0.65 mg of selenium.

PEACH: one medium with skin, contains no protein, 1 gram of fiber, 524 I.U of vitamin A, 19 mg of vitamin C, 5.5 mcg of foliate, 0.97 mg of niacin, 193 mg of potassium, 12 mg of phosphorus, 6.9 mg of magnesium, 5 mg of calcium, 0.4 mg of selenium.

STRAWBERRY: 1 cup of whole strawberries contains no protein, 3 grams of fiber, 39 I.U. of vitamin A, 82 mg of vitamin C, 25.5 mcg of foliate, 239 mg of potassium, 27 mg of phosphorus, 20 mg of calcium, 14 mg of magnesium, 1 mg of selenium, 0.55 mg of iron, 0.42 mg of manganese,

TOMATO: one medium, contains 1.05 grams of protein, 1.35 grams of fiber, 2364 I.U of vitamin A, 25 mg of vitamin C, 46 mcg of foliate, 0.94 mg of niacin, 0.1 mg of vitamin B6, 396.7

mg of potassium, 62.7 mg of phosphorus, 22.8 mg of magnesium, 31.9 mg of calcium, 11.4 mg of sodium, 0.51 mg of iron, 0.8 mg of selenium.

WATERMELON: one medium slice contains 1 gram of protein, 1 gram of fiber, 1050 I.U. of vitamin A, 27 mg of vitamin C, 0.57 mg of niacin, 6.33 mcg of foliate, 0.23 mg of vitamin B1, 0.4 mg of vitamin B6, 332 mg of potassium, 31.5 mg of magnesium, 26 mg of phosphorus, 23 mg of calcium, 0.5 mg of iron, 0.3 mg of selenium.

VEGETABLES:

ARTICHOKE: one medium cooked with no added salt, contains 4.2 grams of protein, 5.5 grams of fiber, 425 mg of potassium, 103 mg of phosphorus, 72 mg of magnesium, 54 mg of calcium, and trace amounts of selenium, iron, manganese, copper and zinc.

ASPARAGUS; ½ cup (about 4 spears) cooked with no salt added, contains 2 grams of protein, 1.5 grams of fiber, 144 mg of potassium, 48.5 mg of phosphorus, 18 mg of calcium, 10 mg of sodium, 9 mg of magnesium,

BROCCOLI: ½ cooked with no added salt, contains 2.3 grams of protein, 2.3 grams of fiber, 228 mg of potassium, 46 mg of phosphorus, 36 mg of calcium, 28 mg of sodium, 18.7 mg of magnesium, 0.65 mg of iron, 110 mcg of vitamin K, and trace amounts of selenium, manganese, copper and zinc.

CARROTS: ½ cup cooked with no salt added, contains 0.85 grams of protein, 2.6 grams of fiber, 177 mg of potassium, 51.5 mg of sodium, 24 mg of calcium, 23.4 mg of phosphorus, 10 mg of magnesium, 0.48 mg of iron, trace amounts of selenium, manganese, copper, and zinc.

CAULIFLOWER; ½ cup cooked with no salt added, contains 1.1 grams of protein, 1.7 grams of fiber, 88 mg of potassium, 19.8 mg of phosphorus, 9.9 mg of calcium, 9.3 mg of sodium, 5.6 mg of magnesium, trace amounts of selenium, copper, iron, manganese, and zinc.

CORN: one ear cooked with no salt added, contains 2.6 grams of protein, 2.1 grams of fiber, 191.7 mg of potassium, 79 mg of phosphorus, 24.6 mg of magnesium, 13 mg of sodium, 1.5 mg of calcium, 0.6 mg of selenium, 0.5 mg of iron, 0.4 mg of zinc.

CUCUMBER: ½ a cup with skin sliced, contains 0.36 grams of protein, 0.42 grams of fiber, 74,9 mg of potassium, 1.4 mg of phosphorus, 5.7 mg of magnesium, 1 mg of sodium, 7.3 mg of calcium, trace amounts of selenium, copper, iron, manganese, and zinc.

GREEN PEPPER: 1 small raw contains 0.66 grams of protein, 1.3 grams of fiber, 14 mg of potassium, 7.4 mg of magnesium, 6.7 mg of calcium, 1.48 mg of sodium.

KALE: 1 cup of cooked with no salt added, contains 2.5 grams of protein, 2.6 grams of fiber, 296 mg of potassium, 36 mg of phosphorus, 23 mg of magnesium, 32 mg of calcium, 29.9 mg of sodium, 1.2 mg of iron, 0.5 mg of manganese, 1.2 mg of selenium, 1062 mcg of vitamin K.

LIMA BEANS: 1 cup of cooked large lima beans with no salt added, contains 14.7 grams of protein, 13.2 grams of fiber, 965 mg of potassium, 208.7 mg of phosphorus, 8.8 mg of magnesium, 32 mg of calcium, 8.5 mg of selenium, 4.5 mg of iron, 3.8 mg of sodium, 1.8 mg of zinc, 0.8 mg of manganese, 0.44 mg of copper.

MUSHROOMS: ½ cup of raw contains 1 gram of protein, 0.42 grams of fiber, 129.5 mg of potassium, 36.4 mg of phosphorus, 3.5 mg of magnesium, 3 mg of selenium, 1.8 mg of calcium, 1.4 mg of sodium, 0.36 mg of iron.

ONIONS: 1 small cooked without salt added, contains 0.8 grams of protein, 1.3 grams of fiber, 110 mg of potassium, 23 mg of phosphorus, 14 mg of calcium, 7 mg of magnesium, 2.1 mg of sodium, 0.42 mg of selenium.

PEAS: 1 cup boiled with no salt added contains 8.58 grams of protein, 8.8 grams of fiber, 433.6 mg of potassium, 187 mg of phosphorus, 62 mg of magnesium, 43 mg of calcium, 4.8 mg of sodium, 2.5 mg of iron, 3 mg of selenium, 1.9 mg of zinc, 0.8 mg of manganese.

POTATOES: 1 medium baked with no salt added, contains 3 grams of protein, 2.3 grams of fiber, 610 mg of potassium, 78 mg of phosphorus, 39 mg of magnesium, 7.8 mg of calcium, 7.8 mg of sodium, 0.55 mg of iron, 0.46 mg of selenium, 0.45 mg of zinc.

SPINACH: one cup of uncooked contains 0.86 grams of protein, 0.81 grams of fiber, 167 mg of potassium, 14.7 mg of phosphorus, 23.7 mg of magnesium, 29.7 mg of calcium, 23.7 mg of sodium, 145 mcg of vitamin K.

SQUASH, SUMMER, ZUCCHINI, one cup of sliced without salt, contains 1.65 grams of protein, 2.5 grams of fiber, 345.6 mg of potassium, 7 mg of phosphorus, 43 mg of magnesium, 48.6 mg of calcium, 1.8 mg of sodium, 0.65 mg of iron, 0.38 mg of manganese, 0.36 mg of selenium, 0.7 mg of zinc.

SQUASH, WINTER: one cup of cubed, baked with no salt added, contains 1.02 grams of protein, 2.07 grams of fiber, 181 mg of potassium, 21.7 mg of phosphorus, 17 mg of magnesium,

32.5 mg of calcium, 27.9 mg of sodium, 0.52 mg of iron, 0.46 mg of selenium,

SWEET POTATOES: one medium, baked in its own skin, contains 1.96 grams of protein, 3.42 grams of fiber, 273 mg of potassium, 29.5 mg of phosphorus, 13.5 mg of magnesium, 6.2 mg of calcium, 11 mg of sodium, 0.55 mg of iron, 0.5 mg of selenium, .06 mg of manganese, 0.3 mg of zinc.

The nutritional values are just approximate and just to acquaint you with the over all values of the most common foods that are consumed. Knowledge of such nutritional values helps us to diversify our meal menus for the optimal intake of right amounts of various foods in conjunction with the supplements we take on a daily basis, either voluntarily or through prescriptions.

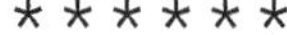

APPENDIX 10

RECOMMENDED NUTRITION INTAKE & THE SOURCES

VITAMIN A

10,000 I.U. (plant derived) per day are recommended for adult males, and 8,000 I.U. for adult females (12,000 I.U. if lactating). Vitamin A helps in cell reproduction, it stimulates immune system, and is required for the formation of some hormones. It helps our vision, bone growth, development of teeth, healthy skin, hair, and mucous membranes. It has been identified to affect prevention against measles. Vitamin A deficiency can cause night blindness, dry skin, poor bone growth, and poor tooth enamel. Beta carotene, alpha carotene and retinol are versions of vitamin A. A significant amount of vitamin A can be sourced from cantaloupes, tomatoes, oranges, kiwi, peaches, watermelon, blackberries, sweet potatoes, kale, green peppers, summer squash (zucchini), carrots, spinach, avocado, asparagus, peas, and broccoli.

Deficiency of vitamin-A can cause deformation of bones, dryness of skin, vision problems including blindness, respiratory infections, etc.

VITAMIN B-1(thiamine):
1.2 mg for adult males and 1.1 mg for females (1.5 mg if lactating) are recommended for consumption each day. Vitamin B-1 (thiamine) helps the body to convert carbohydrates in our food to energy. Therefore, it is important for the production of energy in our body. It is essential for functioning of the heart muscles, and the nervous system. Most fruits and vegetables are not sufficient in thiamin. Its deficiency can cause fatigue and general weakness in our body. It is available in varied quantities in peas, avocado, and watermelon.

Insufficiency or lack of vitamin B-1 can cause heart failure, and muscle weakness.

VITAMIN B-2 (riboflavin):
1.3 mg for adult males and 1.1 mg for females (1.5 mg if pregnant or lactating) are recommended for consumption each day. Vitamin B-2 is important for the body growth, and the reproduction of red cells. It helps in releasing energy from the carbohydrates. Most fruits and vegetables are not a significant source of this vitamin. Kiwi and avocado contain some quantities of this vitamin.

Insufficiency of vitamin B-2 can cause anemia, itchy and red eyes, dry and sore throat, swollen skin, etc.

VITAMIN B-3 (niacin):
16 mg for adult males and 14 mg for women (17 to 18 mg if pregnant or lactating) are recommended for consumption each day. Vitamin B-3 is important for the conversion of food to energy. It assists in the functioning of the digestive system and nerves. It also aids the health of skin. Prominent sources of this vitamin are corn, artichoke, asparagus, summer squash (zucchini), lima beans, sweet potatoes, kale, broccoli, carrots, green peppers, peanuts, pine nuts, chestnuts, and almonds.

Insufficiency of vitamin B-3 can cause diarrhea, skin rashes, disorientation, etc.

VITAMIN B-5 (pantothenic acid)
5 mg for adult men and women (6 to 7 mg for women who are pregnant or lactating) are recommended for consumption on daily basis. It is essential for the metabolism of food in the body. Also, it is essential for the production of hormones, and the good cholesterol. Oranges, bananas, avocado, sweet potatoes, potatoes, corn, lima beans, winter squash, artichokes, mushrooms, broccoli, cauliflower, and carrots, are good sources of this vitamin.

Insufficiency of vitamin B-5 causes tingling in hands and feet, fatigue, headaches, drowsiness, muscle weakness, and infections in some cases.

VITAMIN B-6 (pyridoxine)
1.3 mg to 1.7 mg for male and female adults (2 mg for women who are pregnant or lactating) are recommended for daily consumption. Vitamin B-6 is required for the chemical reaction of proteins. Higher the protein is consumed then higher the need for vitamin B-6 becomes. It plays an important role in the creation of antibodies in the immune system, and also acts in the formation of red blood cells. Besides, it helps to maintain normal nerve function. Good sources of this vitamin are watermelon, bananas, avocado, peas, potatoes, and carrots.

Deficiency of vitamin B-6 causes convulsions, dizziness, nerve damage, skin rashes, irritability, and nausea.

VITAMIN B-7 (biotin)
30 mcg to 100 mcg for adult males and females, and pregnant/lactating women are recommended. Along with other vitamin B s, biotin helps convert food in to energy. For healthy hair, skin,

and nails it is especially important. Good sources of biotin are soy beans, broccoli, sweet potatoes, sunflower seeds, and some nuts.

Deficiency of vitamin B-7 causes split hair, hair loss, weight loss, muscle pain dry and scaly skin, skin rashes, broken nails, etc.

VITMIN B-9 (foliate / folic acid)

400 mcg for male and female adults (500 mcg to 600 mcg for pregnant/lactating women) are recommended for daily consumption. Healthy nails, hair, skin, mucous membranes, nerves, and blood depend on vitamin B-9. Foliate/folic acid is essential for the production of red blood cells, as well as, components of nervous system. Also, it helps in the creation and formation process of RNA and DNA. It is a critical part of spinal fluid. It is important for the maintenance of brain function. It is absolutely essential for proper cell growth and the development of embryo. Women who are pregnant are recommended to take foliate/folic acid in sufficient quantities on daily basis. Prominent sources of this vitamin are: kiwi, blackberries, tomatoes, oranges, strawberries, bananas, cantaloupe, lima beans, asparagus, avocado, peas, artichoke, spinach, winter squash, broccoli, summer squash (zucchini), corn, sweet potatoes, kale, potatoes, carrots, onions, green peppers, peanuts, sunflower seeds, chestnuts, walnuts, hazelnuts, and pine nuts, etc.

Insufficiency of vitamin B-9 causes loss of appetite, weight loss, weakness, swollen tongue, heart palpitations, diarrhea, etc.

VITAMIN B-12

2.4 mcg for male and female adults and 2.6 to 2.8 mcg for pregnant and lactating women are recommended for daily consumption. Like other B vitamins, it is important for our metabolism. Vitamin B-12 helps in the formation of red blood cells, and in the maintenance of central nervous system of the body. The only known sources of this vitamin are fish, meat, poultry, and dairy products.

Deficiency of vitamin B-12 can cause dementia, memory loss, loss of balance, and some neurological problems, etc. Deficiency is quite common among older women.

VITAMIN C

60 mg for male and female adults, 70 mg for pregnant women, and 95 mg for those who are lactating are recommended for daily consumption. This is among the important vitamins in providing protection to the body. It plays a significant role as an antioxidant, and protects the body tissue from the damage of oxidation. Body's metabolism's byproduct free radicals are potentially damaging. Free radicals can cause cell damage which, in turn, contributes to cardio vascular disease (CVD) and cancer. As an antioxidant, vitamin C protects the body from these free radicals. Vitamin C is also an affective anti-viral agent. Prominent sources of this vitamin are: tomatoes, lime, peach, bananas, apples, lemon, grapes, cucumber, green peppers, kale, lima beans, mushrooms, onions, peas, potatoes, spinach, summer squash (zucchini), winter squash, and sweet potatoes.

Lack of vitamin C can lead to a variety of health problems like bleeding gums, loosening of teeth, anemia, general weakness, muscle pain, and various infections.

VITAMIN D

5 mg for male and female adults, 10 mg for male and female adults between 50 years and 70 years, and 15 mg for adults above 70 years. Our bodies manufacture this vitamin after being exposed to sun for about 15 minutes. Vitamin D is vital to the body, and without this calcium and magnesium do not get absorbed by the body. Calcium and phosphorus are essential for the development of healthy bones and teeth, and therefore vitamin D becomes

crucial to their proper absorption and maintenance of balance. Recent research shows that vitamin D is a lot more important than its currently known role of aiding absorption of calcium and magnesium. It is advisable to take adequate dosages of this vitamin, especially if you are above the age of 50.

Deficiency of vitamin D leads to loss of bone mass, cancer, and is linked to many diseases.

VITAMIN E

30 I.U. of male and female adults is recommended for daily consumption. Just like vitamin C, this vitamin also acts like antioxidant to protect body tissues the damage caused by oxidation. It prevents free radicals from damaging cells and tissues. In this way, vitamin E deters atherosclerosis and accelerates wound healing. It helps to minimize the wrinkles, heals minor wounds, and soothes the broken or stressed skin tissue. It plays an important role in the formation of red blood cells and the absorption of vitamin K. Prominent sources of this vitamin are: blackberries, bananas, apples, kiwi, almonds, sunflower seeds, pine, peanuts, and Brazil nuts.

Insufficiency of vitamin-E causes anemia, muscle weakness, slow healing of wounds, dry hair and skin, bruising, nerve damage, etc.

VITAMIN K

70 mcg to 80 mcg for male adults, and 60 mcg to 65 mcg for female adults are recommended for daily consumption. It is needed to form essential proteins, for blood coagulation, kidney function, and bone metabolism. Prominent sources of this vitamin are: spinach, turnip greens, broccoli, cabbage, kale, and other leafy vegetables, pine nuts, cashew nuts, chestnuts, and hazelnuts.

Insufficiency of vitamin-K leads to reduced blood coagulation.

PROTEIN

Protein is an essential nutrient for the body. Protein is required to make new tissue, to grow it, maintain it, and repair it as and when required. Protein is made of a variety of Amino Acids. Some of these amino acids cannot be made by your body and, therefore, must be received through the diet. Protein deficiency causes retarded growth, and also the lack of sufficient protein results in slow healing ability. Meat, poultry, fish, and dairy products are the non vegetarian sources of protein. Beans, lentils grains, nuts, tofu, seeds, and dairy products are the vegetarian sources of protein in our diet. Please note that most vegetables contain some protein, even though the quantity is insignificant. Protein from animal source is concentrated, while the protein from agricultural source is less concentrated. About 0.8 grams of protein for every 2.2 lbs of your body weight is more than enough. Excess amounts of protein cause heavy burden on the liver and kidneys.

MINERALS

CALCIUM

1000 mg for male and female adults are recommended for daily consumption. Calcium helps in the absorption of nutrients through the cell walls. It helps us to sleep, and tend to ease up the insomnia condition. Calcium deficiency can cause difficulties in the contraction of muscles, failure of nerves to carry messages, and clotting of blood, muscle spasms, cramps, etc. Under calcium deficient conditions, the body takes calcium from the bones, which makes the bones weaker and brittle. Brittle bones can beak easily. For seniors, it becomes very important to maintain adequate levels of calcium in the food intake, as this is the time when osteoporosis sets in if the body is denied of calcium. Prominent sources of calcium are: orange, blackberries, kiwi, tomatoes, lime, strawberries, lemon, grapes, apples, cantaloupe, bananas, peach, artichoke, peas, summer squash, broccoli, kale, lima beans, winter squash, spinach, carrots, avocado, asparagus, almonds,

Brazil nuts, pistachio nuts, walnuts, chestnuts, macadamia nuts, pecans, sunflower seeds, hazelnuts, cashews, pumpkin seeds, and pine nuts etc.

COPPER

1.3 mg to 3 mg per day for male and female adults is recommended. Copper helps in the absorption, metabolism, and storage of iron in our bodies. It also helps in the supply of oxygen to the body, as well as in the formation process of red blood cells. Copper deficiency will cause lack of iron, and will result in anemia. Prominent sources of copper are: apples, bananas, blackberries, cantaloupe, grapes, kiwi lemon, lime, orange, peach, strawberry, tomatoes, lima beans, artichoke, avocado, broccoli, carrots, cauliflower, corn, cucumber, green peppers, kale, mushrooms, onions, peas, potatoes, spinach, summer and winter squash, and sweet potatoes, etc.

IODINE

150 mcg per day for male and female adults, 175 mcg per day for pregnant women are recommended. Iodine promotes healthy hair, skin, nails, and teeth. For centuries, it has been known to prevent goiter, as a part of several thyroid hormones, it strongly influences nutrient metabolism, nerve and muscle function. Its deficiency in the body may cause weight gain, hair loss, insomnia, and some forms of mental retardation. Prominent sources of this mineral are: kelp, and vegetables and nuts grown in iodine rich soil.

IRON

15 mg for adult females, 10 mg for adult males, and 30 mg for pregnant women are recommended for daily consumption. There are two kinds of dietary iron. Heme iron is found in animal products and non-heme iron which is found in dark green vegetables, grains, nuts, and dried fruits. Non-heme iron, derived from non animal source is best absorbed when consumed with vitamin C. Nuts, fruits and vegetables containing iron should

be consumed simultaneously with vitamin C to obtain the best results. An important aspect to note is that vitamin E should be taken separately with an interval because if taken with iron, its affects will be neutralized. If you are a complete vegetarian, then you may require an extra dose of iron in natural form or in supplement form. Prominent sources of iron are: blackberries, kiwi, strawberries, tomatoes, bananas, grapes, lima beans, peas, avocado, kale, spinach, broccoli, summer squash, potatoes, sweet potatoes, winter squash, corn, carrots, mushrooms, and a small amount in most nuts.

MAGNESIUM

320 mg to 420 mg per day for adult females and males are recommended. It is an important ingredient of bone. It is essential for healthy bones, teeth, and reduces the risk of developing osteoporosis. Adequate levels of magnesium in the blood stream protect the body from cardio vascular disease (CVD) and stroke. Need for magnesium increases with the incidence of stress and illness in the body. As a supplement, under medical advice, it can successfully treat insomnia, muscle cramps, premenstrual syndrome, high blood pressure, angina, leg cramps due to poor blood circulation, cardio vascular disease (CVD) heart disease, stroke, and increase the chances for survival among stroke and heart attack patients. It is needed for making new cells, activating B vitamins, relaxing nerves and muscles, energy production, and in clotting blood. It also helps in the absorption of calcium, potassium, and vitamin C. Magnesium deficiency could cause fatigue, muscle weakness, heart problem, high blood pressure, insomnia, osteoporosis, and nervousness. Prominent sources of Magnesium are: kiwi, bananas, tomatoes, blackberries, strawberries, oranges, avocado, artichoke, peas, summer squash, potatoes, corn, spinach, kale, broccoli, winter squash, sweet potatoes, Brazil nuts, cashews, almonds, pumpkin seeds, pine nuts, peanuts, walnuts, macadamia nuts, pecans, sunflower seeds, pistachios, chestnuts, and hazelnuts, etc.

MANGANESE

2 to 5 mg per day for male and female adults is recommended. It is essential for proper formation and maintenance of bones, cartilages, and connective tissues. It acts as an antioxidant, and assists in normal blood coagulation. It functions in enzyme reactions, thyroid hormone function, blood sugar, and metabolism. Most prominent sources of manganese are: blackberries, strawberries, peas, lima beans, sweet potatoes, kale, summer squash, pine nuts, pecans, walnuts, and chestnuts, etc.

PHOSPHORUS

800 mg per day for male and female adults (1200 mg for pregnant women) are recommended. Like calcium, it is necessary for the formation of bones, nerve cells, and teeth. Phosphorus deficiency, though rare, cause loss of appetite, general weakness, and bone pain. Prominent sources of this mineral are: kiwi, tomatoes, blackberries, bananas, strawberries, orange, peach, lime, cantaloupe, lima beans, peas, artichoke, avocado, corn, potatoes, asparagus, broccoli, kale, mushrooms, sweet potatoes, sunflower seeds, brazil nuts, cashews, pine nuts, pistachios, almond, peanuts, walnuts, chestnuts, pecans, macadamia nuts, hazelnuts, and pumpkin seeds, etc.

POTASSIUM

2000 mg per day for adult females and males is recommended. It is essential to maintain fluid balance, growth, and regulation of heart beat and blood pressure. It is also required for carbohydrate metabolism, insulin secretion by the pancreas, and protein synthesis. Studies suggest that people who regularly consume potassium rich foods are less likely to develop atherosclerosis, high blood pressure, heart disease, or to die of a stroke. Deficiency may cause muscle cramps, high blood pressure, heart disease, stroke, irregular heart beat, insomnia and kidney and lung failure. Prominent sources of potassium are: bananas, tomatoes, blackberries, strawberry, orange, cantaloupe, peach, grapes, apples, lemon, lime, avocado, lima beans, potatoes, peas, artichokes, summer squash, kale, sweet potatoes, broccoli, corn, winter squash, spinach, asparagus, green peppers, mushrooms, onions, cauliflower, cucumber, chestnuts, sunflower seeds, pistachios, almonds, brazil nuts, peanuts, cashews, pine nuts, walnuts, pecans, macadamia nuts, and hazelnuts, etc.

SELENIUM

70 mcg per day for male adults, 55 mcg for female adults, and 65 mcg for pregnant women are recommended. It is an antioxidant which protects cells and tissues from damage by free radicals. It supports the immune system, and works in conjunction with vitamin E. Adequate levels of selenium may prevent stroke, heart disease, arthritis, and cancer. Its prominent sources are: bananas, kiwi, strawberries, blackberries, tomatoes, orange peach, apples, grape, lima beans, peas, mushroom, kale, corn, sweet potatoes, winter squash, onions, summer squash, spinach, Brazil nuts, sunflower seeds, cashews, pistachios, peanuts, walnuts, almonds, chestnuts, and pecans.

SODIUM

500 mg per day for female and male adults is recommended. All body fluids, including blood, tears, perspiration, etc. contain sodium. It regulates the blood volume and pressure, and maintains optimal pH levels. High sodium levels in the body deplete potassium, and cause the body to retain water, which causes the blood pressure to rise. A low sodium diet can reduce the high blood pressure and correct the potassium deficiency. However, overexertion can cause temporary sodium deficiency, and present symptoms of nausea, dehydration, muscle cramps, and other symptoms of stroke or heart attack. Sodium occurs in almost all fruits, vegetables, and nuts. Peanuts, pumpkin seeds, cashews, pistachios, chestnuts, macadamia nuts, and almonds do contain significant amounts.

ZINC

15 mg daily for male and female adults, 30 mg per day for pregnant women are recommended. It is integral to synthesis of RNA and DNA, the genetic material that controls cell growth, cell division, and cell function. It contributes to many body processes like: metabolism, wound healing, liver's ability to remove toxic substances, immune system, regulates the heart rate and blood pressure, Adequate zinc levels promote healthy skin and hair, short term memory and attention span. Deficiency of zinc can cause stunted growth; poor wound healing, white spots on the nails, hair loss, and fatigue. On the other hand, too much of zinc in the body can impair the immune system and produce symptoms like vomiting, fatigue, kidney problems, and stomach ache. Once again, balance is the key.

For clean arteries and adequate blood circulation, certain practices can be of immense help to our maintaining a healthy body. If onions, garlic, ginger, cayenne peppers, paprika, lime, whole grains, beans, lentils, olive oil, fat free milk, hard tofu, a variety of vegetables and fruits covering all ranges of color, oat bran and wheat bran, green or processed tea, and maintaining a healthy life style under non toxic environment are not a part of your current daily life then make every effort to incorporate them in anything and everything you eat.

For example, unless you happen to like the taste of ***GARLIC***, and are used to its regular use in your meals, you will find it a bit strong. Consumption of raw garlic leaves a garlic odor in mouth for several hours. Just live with it, or alternatively, let the garlic cook along with the food, in which case the garlic will not have any residual odor. Garlic is a member of onion family of plants, and it has been a part of daily food of peoples around the world for thousands of years. Also, it has been considered a medicinal plant in many cultures who considered it to possess healing properties. Garlic has sulfur containing compounds with biological activity, with numerous benefits. Some of the most beneficial effects of garlic are on Cardio Vascular System. Its regular consumption can lower the blood pressure tremendously. Additionally, it lowers the blood cholesterol and blood fats (triglycerides). It increased the supply of the good cholesterol (HDL). It also stops the bad cholesterol (LDL) to get oxidized. LDL oxidization causes damage to the arterial walls. Garlic offers a noticeable protection against the cardio vascular disease (CVD). Garlic is also an antiseptic and an antibiotic which discourage the growth of many kinds of bacteria and fungi in the body. It enhances the immune system by increasing the number of killer cells that check the spread of many diseases. It contains antioxidant compounds which makes garlic to protect liver and the brain cells from degenerative changes. It also lowers blood sugar.

There is another very important food item and that is ***GINGER*** which has been popular as a food as well as a medicine for thousands of years in older cultures. When consumed, it provides a warming effect and helps the digestion. It settles upset stomach, and relieves pain. It contains antioxidants and enzymes, and produces a boosting effect that boosts digestion of proteins, and protects against intestinal parasites and motion sickness. It is known to improve the blood circulation, and provides protection against cancer causing agents that can mutate the DNA.

There are a variety of ***HERBS*** that can prove to be beneficial to you. In spite of all the good guidance, women are suggested to use these herbs in less than recommended quantities, just to see if they are workable and beneficial. All herbs have a long list of nutritional values which can be of real benefit to all women, however, they should be consumed in small quantities, so that not to allow too much nutrition concentration of one kind to suffocate the digestive system.

* * * * * *

APPENDIX 11

YOGURT

The recommendation of yogurt has been repeated several times in this book, because it is probably the most beneficial food there is. This food is absolutely natural in every sense of the word. In making yogurt specific bacteria strains are introduced in to the warm milk which then ferments under the controlled temperature for a few hours. The bacteria ingest the natural lactose and release lactic-acid as a waste product (poop). The acidity from lactic acid makes the milk to curdle in to a texture which yogurt has. This acidity is about 4.5 pH, and it promotes the growth of beneficial bacteria like: ***lactobacillus bulgaricus, streptococcus, thermophilus, and lactobacillus acidophilus.***

Benefits of eating yogurt on daily basis are numerous, and more will be discovered in the years to follow. Some of the benefits are:

*contains 13 grams, protein, 590 mgs of potassium, 452 mgs of calcium in 1 cup.
*it restores the gut flora

*protects against unhealthy organisms in the gut and vagina
*reestablishes the population of good bacteria which get destroyed by the use of antibiotics
*helps in the treatment of a variety of gastrointestinal conditions
*prevents antibiotic associated diarrhea

*boosts immune system and prevents infections
*reduces vaginal yeast infection
*provides relief from indigestion
*controls growth of fungus in candida infection
*binds anti-carcinogen substances and prevents colon cancer
*lowers cholesterol levels in the bloodstream, and reduced the risk of heart disease
*contains easily absorbable calcium and reduces the risk of osteoporosis

*provides relief from constipation
*clears up symptoms of colitis, inflammatory bowel syndrome, bowel disease
*fights and prevents urinary tract and bladder infections,
*helps the body to make family of vitamin B vitamin in the intestines
*reduces estrogen hormones in women thereby minimizing various cancer risks
*stops anal itching
*reduces symptoms of lactose intolerance
*reduces response related to inflammation and hypersensitivity, etc.

⋆ ⋆ ⋆ ⋆ ⋆ ⋆

APPENDIX 12

OMEGA 6 AND OMEGA 3

There are two families of fatty acids that are essential to the body, which are omega 6 and omega 3. They are important components of cell membranes to maintain flexibility and keep it fluid. They are the building blocks of chemical messengers, known as ***postaglandins***, which regulate the cardiovascular system, brain, flexibility of joints, fat, protective response to inflammation, metabolism, skin health, ad nervous system.

Omega 6 controls and lowers the cholesterol in the bloodstream, including HDL which is good cholesterol, promotes blood clotting, increases the blood pressure, and increases the oxidation of LDL, the bad cholesterol, if consumed in excess. High levels of omega 6 in the body may not be good for most women, because ***Arachidonic Acids*** (**AA**) (Trans Fatty Acids) are found in it, which tend to cling to the inside of the arterial walls and cause blockages. Also, it causes inflammation.

Eicosapentaenoic Acid (**EPA**) is a part of ***omega 3*** which cleans the inside walls of arteries and is non-inflammatory but in excess it may be abrasive and cause scarring. Omega 3 decreases the sub-class of small particles of LDL (bad cholesterol), and reduces the chances of sudden cardiac death. It is anti-clotting, anti-diabetic, and anti-depressant; lowers lipoprotein, and reduces the inflammation in the coronary plaque. Omega 3 lowers the ***triglycerides*** (three fatty acids) which are large molecules of fatty substance. This is the fat which is stored in the body, and gets accumulated in our body through consumption of vegetable and animal fats, and carbohydrates. Some fat is good for the body, and it should be around 10% of the body weight.

Women with high triglycerides have lower HDL (good cholesterol) and high levels of LDL (bad cholesterol). Lower the triglycerides the better it is. Omega 3 in an optimal ratio to omega 6 lowers triglycerides.

Both fats are good for the body and cannot be inter-changed, and both should be consumed in an optimal ratio to each other. The optimal ratio of Omega 6 and Omega 3 is 3:1, (3 grams of Omega 6 to 1 gram of Omega 3), and both are available with varying ratios in vegetable sources like soy milk, berries, peas, flaxseed oil, beans, tofu, flaxseeds, walnuts, and canola oil, etc.

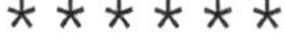

APPENDIX 13

GENES

Genetic science is an emerging science and the potential of breakthroughs in healing are more than what current researchers can handle. They have yet to agree with each other as to the number of genes in a human cell. The estimates range from 19,000 to 80,000 genes, however, quite many researchers, including Dr. Peter D'Adamo, seem to agree with number to be around 30,000. At this time, it is known that there are 6,000 genes in Fungi, 19,000 genes in most Worms, 30,000 in most humans, 40,000 in Fish, and 60,000 in most plants, and many more estimates of genes have yet to be discovered in millions of other species.

Like any other species, genes in cells adapt themselves in response to the environment, food, nutrition, toxins, bacterial and viral invasions, hot and cold temperatures, etc. As a result, some genes are suppressed while others flourish, even when we were in the womb. At other times, in certain environment, the previously suppressed genes become active and fully functional. Each gene is specifically programmed to perform certain function/s.

According to Matt Ridley in his book 'Genome', DNA is not only structurally important but also functionally active substances which determine the biochemical activities and specific characteristics of cells. Genes in cells carry information from the very beginning, before the plant life, from a mere cell form to the current state of humans. The genes in your body have genetic codes from the beginning of human evolution and all the developmental steps in between.

Comparatively, Humans are 98% Chimpanzees and Chimpanzees are 98% Humans. Chimpanzees are 97% Gorillas and Humans are 97% Gorillas. Humans are more Chimpanzees than Gorillas. About 75% Chicken genes and more than 88% genes of Rats, Mice, Swine, and most birds are identical to human genes. They are close relatives of all humanity. As Erasmus Darwin, grandfather of Charles Darwin, said in 1794 that the filament of life is the same as has ever been for all life forms which are almost similar to each other……

Researchers have been able to identify specific diseases with specific chromosomes. Breast cancer, Alzheimer's disease with chromosome 1, small cell lung cancer to chromosome 3, diabetes mellitus to chromosome 5, lung cancer and obesity to chromosome 12, pancreatic cancer to chromosome 13, so and so forth.

Speedy research in genes is unraveling so many genetic therapies and cures that it is hard to keep up with the news. In genetic code there are 'restrictive enzymes' that can cut a viral DNA and glue it in a non-viral combination, called recombinant DNA. In this way many or all diseases can be cured.

For example, researchers have identified APOE gene with E2, E3, and E4 versions. Women with E4 gene are at a higher risk of getting heart disease, and women with two E4 genes are predisposed to heart disease. It was also determined that E4 gene appears mostly in white people from North European origin, blacks from Africa, Polynesians, and people from New Guinea. Also, E4 has been linked to diet of meats and fatty foods. Genetic tests can reveal who should stop eating meat and fats, and who can.

E4 gene plays a key role in Alzheimer's disease which was earlier linked to nickel pots and pans, aluminum, arterial plaque, etc, but today it is linked to E4. Many researchers say "All Disease is genetic ". The culprit gene is E4 and its bad version in families causes Alzheimer's risk factor from 20% to 90%, depending upon age. If you have two E4 genes then your chances of getting Alzheimer's are very high.

E4 effects are more severe in women than men. **More women have Alzheimer's than men worldwide**. E3 is known to reduce the risk, however women with E4 and E3 genes (one culprit and one good) are at higher risk than men with E4 and E4 (2 culprit genes).

E4 version of APOE gene tends to stimulate build up of ***Amyloid Beta Peptide*** (a protein which becomes plaque) inside the neurons of Alzheimer's patients. For some unknown reasons, E4 version helps the growth of this destructive plaque (Amyloid Beta Peptide). There is another gene, SORL 1, which has been found linked to Amyloid plaque build up in the brain. Amyloid is a toxic protein and both of these genes cause it to grow excessively.

Whether science bends toward cloning humans or not, it has yet to be found out in coming years, but it is a fact that it is possible now. This could raise ethical, legal, political, and religious questions which will require new laws, their passage, and acceptance. However, in the meantime, there is a very happy marriage between science and conventional cures. Research shows that women who for example have genes that make them susceptible to getting bowel cancer, a regular diet of Aspirin and unripe bananas may be the ideal cure. Here, genetic science identifies and diagnoses the problem which can be cured with conventional measures, a good example for an acceptable and functional cooperation.

Genes in anyone's body are constantly coping and improvising in response to internal and external environmental challenges. For millions of years genes have evolved, progressed, and adapted to changing environment each step of the evolutionary process. Even today when there is a hundred fold polluted environment, genes have adapted to it for the time being but not without marked signs of identifiable negative impact.

To a significant extent genes are the blueprint of several physiological events in human life path. I strongly believe that even thoughts, emotions, behavior, dreams, and other non-physiological events in human life are influenced by genes. By improving our lifestyle, health, emotions, behavior, thoughts, deeds, etc., we not only improve our life events in the near future but also sow the genetic seeds that will positively affect the health and mindset of our off springs and the generations thereafter.

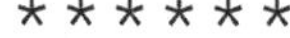

APPENDIX 14

EXERCISE

For the past decade or two we have been talking a lot about the importance of exercise for good health and wellness. There are marked benefits of exercising on a regular basis, but there are some side effects of it also with varying degrees.

Among the benefits, we have experienced that exercise increases the blood circulation, pumps oxygen in the lungs for cleansing the blood, maintains the pumping of heart and its muscles working, uses the calcium and other minerals which are important for bone health, stimulates the organs of the body, reinforces and stimulates the cardio vascular system, invigorates strengthens the muscles, generates cell activity in the body areas which are not normally subjected adequate stimulation in our modern and luxurious lifestyle, improves blood circulation in the brain which consumes a significant portion of oxygen and sugar fed in to the body, etc. Light exercising regularly is wonderful for the majority of women.

The flip side of this coin is that vigorous and strenuous exercises can bring out the ever present weaknesses in some organs and other parts of the body as well. Human body grows from a fetus to an adult in an evolutionary process, and not in a mechanical process. Evolutionary process is influenced by internal, external, and genetic influences which have an unlimited array of possibilities and variations. By the time human body reaches adulthood there had been numerous changes in the body, internally and externally. No one comes out with a 'perfect' body which is, in essence, a combination of several systems in a somewhat harmonious partnership. Each of these systems functions differently and therefore is affected differently.

If for some reason the exercise schedule is disrupted for a few days to a few weeks then there lies a high probability of weight gain. Women with a heavy exercising schedule will most likely experience joint pains during the senior years, just like the tennis players experience wrist, elbow, and shoulder related pains; and long distance runners develop knee problems, etc.

There are inherent strengths and weaknesses in the body. When we put this imperfect natural body on a perfect machine which is designed and constructed precisely, we run in to an invisible conflict. If precise measurements are taken, human body will reveal that there are numerous skeletal and muscular imperfections like in shoulders, arms, legs, ears, eyes, etc which don't match up in measurement with each other. Even the pelvic bone is not symmetrical, which bears the heavy pounding in most exercises. This imperfection can be seen almost everywhere in the body. Even the steps taken by our feet have defined differences. When an imperfect human body exercises on a precisely made machine, the outcome cannot be positive for all. Some joints, muscles, and limbs will receive more and unbalanced stress than others. In time, this process will produce skeletal, muscular, and bone joint problems.

Women involved in feverish and strenuous exercise routines will be pulling themselves away from femininity. Feverish and strenuous exercise will develop muscles with male disposition, and increase the level of testosterones in the body. Such women have difficulty in getting pregnant.

High levels of testosterones in women will indicate muscle build up, change in body contours, more body hair than average, deepening of voice, acne (inflammatory disease of sebaceous glands in the skin, which secrete oily substance to lubricate the skin), enlarged clitoris, menstrual irregularity, and frontal balding, decreased fertility, etc. When estrogen levels drop significantly, women face serious risk factors for getting certain cancers, heart disease, stroke, osteoporosis, and bone fractures. On the other hand, abnormally increased levels of estrogen can cause obesity, over weight, high blood pressure, cervical cancer, etc.

Subjecting an imperfect body to a perfect machine at the Gym will most likely develop muscles unevenly and change the natural contours of women. For example, muscles in one arm may look larger and stronger than in other, a layer of muscles may appear on the hips which was not there before, etc and turning women to less feminine, less attractive, and less beautiful.

Regular feverish exercising pushes nutrition to the bones, muscles, and the joints, etc. and in senior years when such exercises are not possible, the nutrition, especially calcium and other minerals will get deposited in the joints resulting in excruciating joint pains requiring surgery. Also, prolonged and feverish exercise routine programs the body to keep routing the nutrition to the bones and joints even after such exercising has been stopped, causing excessive calcium and mineral build up in some bones and joints, thereby creating an environment for arthritis to develop. Among many types of arthritis, infectious arthritis can be very painful, which is caused by ***gonococcus*** bacterium that causes gonorrhea.

Also knee joints attract ***staphylococcus, streptococcus***, and ***pneumococcus*** which are linked to meningitis, pneumonia, and various abscesses.

Additionally, strenuous exercise brings out the inherent weaknesses in muscles, joints, organs, bones, and vascular system, etc. which were not causing any problems before. Fatigue and endurance capacities of the vital components of human body have different breaking points, and they don't need to be tested just to feel good.

Exercising should be light, regular, involving all body parts through diverse body functions, not punishing, not disturbing the natural hormonal balance, interesting and useful, maintaining the essence of femininity, and which can be carried out easily to the old age without breaking the routine.

According to Elin Ekblom-Bak of Swedish School of Sport and Health Sciences, exercise should be spread throughout the day and not concentrated in very small time zone. People who sit most of the day and exercise in the gymnasium for an hour are not receiving the full benefits of exercising. In fact, sitting more than 3 to 4 hours in one place may make you fat, cause heart attack, or even death. In this context, Elin Ekblom-Bak explains that sitting for longer periods can make the genes that regulate the amount of glucose and fat in the body to start sending stress signals and begin to shut down their activity. She believes that doing small things and moving your body throughout the day provide you with meaningful benefits of exercise.

If you have a desk job then make sure that you get up at the slightest excuse like speaking to a colleague, dropping of some inter-office memo, explaining something, in person rather sending an e-mail message or using the phone. Such efforts will momentarily pull you out of sitting position and provide you with some physical activity.

The purpose of any exercise should be to maintain good blood circulation and muscle tone without changing the body contours and feminine beauty which are part of being women.

Prem K. Bhandari, January 2010.

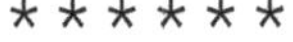

READING REFERENCES

Print Publications

- The Longevity Factor by Joseph Maroon
- The Science of Staying Young by John Morley, Sheri Coberg
- Strong Women Stay Slim by Miriam Nelson
- Evidence of Harm by David Kirby
- Lead Poisoning by Joseph Breen, Cindy Stoup
- Inflammation Nation by Floyd Chilton, Laura Tucker
- Beating Diabetes by David Nathan, Linda Delahanty
- Diabetes by Paula Ford-Martin
- The Myth of Alzheimer's by Peter Whitehouse
- Multiple Sclerosis by Rosalind Kalb
- The Migraine Brain by Carolyn Bernstein
- Beautiful Bone without Hormones by Leon Root
- Intestinal Cystitis by Robert Moldwin
- Bone Building Solutions by Sam Grace, Leticia Roa, Carolyn D'Marco

-What if it is not Alzheimer's? By Murray Grossman

-Can't Remember What I Forgot by Sue Halpern

-Breast Cancer Clear and Simple by American Cancer Society

-The Secret History of War on Cancer by Devra Davis

-Understanding Cancer by Norman Coleman

-The Melanoma Book by Howard Kaufman

-What To Eat If You Have Cancer? By Maureen Keene, Daniella Chace

-Abnormal PAP Smears by Nancy Joste

-Uterine Fibroids by Elizabeth Stewart

-Infection Protection by Ronald Klatz, Robert Goldman

-Complete Guide to Colorectal Cancer by American Cancer Society

-What Your Doctor May Not Tell About Colorectal Cancer by Mark Bennett Pochapin

-Bladder Cancer by Derek Raghavan, Kathleen Tuthill,

-Dr. Susan Love's Breast Book by Susan Love

-The Autoimmune Epidemic by Donna Jackson Nakazawa

-Navigating Breast Cancer, Lillie Shockney

-Understanding Cancer Therapies by Helen S.L. Chan

-Living with Cancer by Dave Visel

-Osteoporosis by Arthritis Foundation

-The Human Genome by R. Scott Hawley, Catherine A. Mori

-Genome by Matt Ridley

-The Metabolism Miracle by Diane Kress

-Super Foods by Steven Pratt, Kathy Mathews

-The Sugar Solutions by the Editors of Prevention Magazine, Ann Fittante

-Digestive Wellness by Elizabeth Lipski

-Gut Solutions by Brenda Watson

-Irritable Bowel Syndrome by Rosemary Nicol

-Crohn's Disease and Ulcerative Colitis by Fred Saibil

-Crohn's Disease and Ulcerative Colitis by Jill Sklar

-Diabetes Mellitus by Sue A. Milchovich

-Living with Diabetes by American Medical Association

-Dr Sanjeev Chopra's Liver Book by Sanheev Chopra

-Mayo Clinic's Heart Book

-The Healthy Heart Miracle by Gabe Merkin, Diane Merkin

-Heart Care for Life by Barry Zarret, Genell Subak-Sharpe

-Prescription for Nutritional Health by Phyllis A. Balch

-Healing Immune Disorders by Andrew Gaeddert

-Omega Zone by Barry Sears

-The Atkins Essentials, by Dr. Atkins

-The Microbiotic Path to Total Health by Michio Kushi, Alex Jack

-Strong Women and Men Beat Arthritis by Miriam Nelson

-Breast Cancer by Yashar Hirschaut, Pete Pressman

-Everyone's Guide to Cancer Therapy by Andrew Ko, Malin Dollinger, Ernest Rosenbaum

-The Myth of Osteoporosis by Gillian Samson

-Better Bone Better Body by Susan Brown

-Be a Survivor: Colorectal Cancer by Vladimir Lange

-Gale Encyclopedia of Cancer: Vaginal Cancer by Belinda Rowland

-Skin Cancer by Keyvan Nouri

-Skin Cancer by Po-Lin So

-What you really need to know about Moles and Melanoma by Jill Schofield, William Robinson

-ABC of Skin Cancer by Sajjad Rajpar, Jerry Marsden

-Skin Cancer Recognition and Management by Robert Schwartz

-Lung Cancer by Jack Roth, James Cox, Waun Ki Hong

-How to Survive Lung Cancer by Michael Lloyd

-Papers on Blood Poisoning, Typhoid, Typhus, and other Zymotic Diseases By A. Moffitt

-Preventing and Reversing Osteoporosis by Alan Gaby

-Albanese Bone Loss Causes, Detection, and Therapy by Anthony August Albanese

-Breast Cancer Survival Manual by John Link

-Breast Cancer: The Complete Guide by Jane Brody

-Heal & Prevent Stroke & Heart Disease by Prem K. Bhandari

-The Hygiene System by Herbert Shelton

-Medical Parasitology by Markell Edward and Marietta

-Common ailments by J.H. Oliver

-The Nature Cure Treatment of Varicose Veins and Ulcers by Russell Snedden

-Herbs and Phyto Therapy by Anton Kraak

-The Danger of Food Contamination by Aluminum by Cooper LeHunte

-The Chronic Diseases by Dr. Jain

-Pathological Basis of Diseases by Vinay Kumar, Ramzi Cotran, Stanley Robbins

-Dr. Dean Ornish's Program for Reversing Heart Disease without Drugs And Surgery

-Scientific Documentation as a Basis for the Declaration of Miracles by Canadian Medical Association Journal

-Risk of Ulcerative Colitis among Former and Current Cigarette Smokers By New England Journal of Medicine

-Life Expectancy Following Dietary Modification or Smoking Cessation By S.A. Grover

-Cardiovascular Effects of Omega-3 Fatty Acids by A. Leaf in New England Journal of Medicine

-Omega-3 Fatty Acids and Cancer by R. A. Karmali in Journal of Internal Medicine

-Biological Effects of a Diet of Soy Protein rich in Isoflavones on the Menstrual Cycle of Pre-menopausal Women By A. Cassidy, American Journal of Clinical Nutrition

-Spontaneous Healing by Andrew Weil

-Pancreatic Cancer by Howard A. Reber

-Pancreatic Cancer: Methods and Protocol by Gloria H. Su

-Kidney Stones Handbook by Gail R. Savitz, Stephen W. Leslie

-Enjoying Life with Chronic Obstructive Pulmonary Disease by T.L. Petty, L.M. Nett

-Courage and Information for Life with Chronic Obstructive Pulmonary Disease by R. Carter, B. Nicotra, J.V. Tucker

-Circulation of Blood (Every Man's Library) by William Harvey

-Total Heart Health by Robert H. Schneider, Jeremy Z. Fields

-Heal Your Heart by Joseph C. Piscatella, Barry A. Franklin

* * * * * *

Online Resources

The New England Journal of Medicine www.nejm.com/

Research Medical Library www.mdanderson.org/

Post Graduate Medical Journal www.highwire.stanford.edu/

Medscape Medical News Journal www.medscape.com/

Journal of American Medical Association www.jama.ama-assn.org

British Medical Journal www.bmj.com/

Watch Medical Journal www.jwatch.org/

Sage Journal www.mcr.sagepub.com/

The Calicut Medical Journal www.calicutmedicaljournal.org/

Online Magazines www.onlinenewspapers.com

Healthcare Republic www.healthcarerepublic.com

The Health Journal www.thehealthjournal.com/

MediZine OnLine www.deizine.com/

Prevention Magazine www.prevention.com

Total Health Magazine www.totalhealthmagazine.com

Top Cancer News www.topcancernews.com

Hospital News www.hospitalnews.com/

Healthy Choices www.healthychoices.ca/

Diabetic Lifestyle www.diabetic-lifestyle.com/

Ability Magazine www.abilitymagazine.com/

Indian Journal of Medical Sciences www.indianjmedsci.org/

Nutrition Journal www.nutritionj.com/

Medical Journals (various) www.cancernews.com/

Karger Medical & Scientific Publishers www.karger.com/

Elsevier Medical Publishers www.elsevierhealth.com

Duke University Medical Center www.mclibrary.duke.edu/

Medical Literature www.lungcanceronline.org/

Diagnostic & Interventional Radiology www.dirjournal.org/

Journal of Medical Licensure & Discipline www.journalonline.org

Medical Journals www.unn-edu.net

Phytochemicals: www.pytochemicals.org/

Medical Laboratory Observer www.mlo-online.com/

American Medical Writers Association www.amwa.org/

Indian Bio-Medical Literature www.medindia.nic.in/

Journal of Bio Sciences www.ias.ac.in/biosci/index.html

National Institute of Health www.nih.gov

Center for Disease Control www.cdc.gov

Agency for Healthcare Research and Quality

Breast Cancer	www.breastcancer.org
	www.cancer.gov
	www.breastcancer.about.com
	www.cancer.org/
Esophageal Cancer	www.acidreflux.com
	www.cancer.gov
	www.mayoclinic.com
	www.nlm.nih.gov
	www.gitract.info
	www.cancer.org

Pancreatic Cancer	www.treatingpancreaticcancer.com
	www.cancercenter.com
	www.pancreatic.org
	www.pancan.org
	www.cancer.gov
	www.pancreaticcancer.org.uk
	www.mayoclinic.com
	www.webmed.com
Lung Cancer	www.medicinenet.com
	www.lungcancer.org
	www.cancercenter.com
	www.mayoclinic.com
	www.Emedicinehealth.com
	www.cancer.gov
Skin Cancer	www.webmed.com
	www.skincancer.derma.net
	www.cancer.about.com
	www.aad.org
	www.mayclinic.com
	www.skincancer.org
	www.nih.gov
	www.medicinenet.com
Stomach Cancer	www.acidrefluxlife.com
	www.acidreflux.com
	www.kosmix.com
	www.cancer.net

Cervical Cancer	www.nlm.nih.gov
	www.webmed.com
	www.cervicalcancerfacts.com
	www.cancer.gov
	www.webmed.com
	www.medicinenet.com
	www.mayoclinic.com
	www.cervicalcancer.org
	www.merck.com
Colorectal Cancer	www.medlineplus.gov
	www.avastine.com
	www.cancer.gov
	www.mayclinic.com
	www.cdc.gov
Urinary Bladder Cancer	www.mdanderson.com
	www.medifocus.com
	www.bladderdisorders.info
	www.cancerresearch.com
	www.cancerlinksusa.com/bladder
	www.cancercenter.com
Uterine Cancer	www.uterine-cancer.com
	www.cancercenter.com
	www.medlineplus.gov

Vaginal Cancer	www.nlm.nih.gov
	www.cancer.gov
	www.cancer.org
	www.cancercenter.com
	www.medicinenet.com
	www.mayoclinic.com
	www.moffitt.org
Stroke	www.stroke.org
	www.medicinenet.com
	www.stroke.ahajournal.org
	www.strokeassociation.org
	www.mayoclinic.com
	www.strokecenter.org
	www.healthcenter.com
	www.stroke.about.com
	www.strokeRxInfo.com
Heart Disease	www.americanheart.org
	www.aha.org
	www.heart.org
	www.heartandstroke.ca
	www.heartandstroke.com
	www.cdc.gov
	www.nih.gov
Liver Disease	www.medlineplus.gov
	www.dukehealth.org
	www.medicinenet.com
	www.liver-disease.suite101.com

	www.livermd.org www.righthealth.com
Liver Cancer	www.livercancer.com www.livercancersymptoms.org/ www.aboutlivertumors.com/ www.cancer.gov
Jaundice	www.jaundice.respironics.com www.livestrong.com/jaundice www.medicinenet.com/jaundice/article.htm www.medlineplus.gov
Hepatitis	www.cdc.gov/hepatitis www.medlineplus.gov www.avert.org/hepatitis.htm www.webmed.com/hepatitis/default.htm www.mayoclinic.com
Cirrhosis	www.liverfoundation.org www.nlm.nih.gov www.umm.edu/liver/chronic.htm www.digestive.niddk.nih.gov www.medicinenet.com
Kidney Disease	www.medlineplus.gov www.gwhospital.com www.kidney.org www.webmd.com

	www.emedicinehealth.com
Gallbladder Disease	www.merck.com
	www.womanshealth.about.com
	www.gallbladder.net
	www.mygallbladderinfo.com
	www.cancercenter.com
	www.naturallycuregallstones.com
	www.home-remedies-for-you.com
Intestinal Diseases	www.healthinsite.gov.au
	www.medicinenet.com
	www.healthy.net
	www.cancercenter.com
Crohn's Disease	www.crohnsonline.com
	www.tulane.edu
	www.digestive.niddk.nih.gov
	www.healthy.net
	www.healthinsite.gov.au
Diverticulosis	www.diverticulosis.net
	www.medicinenet.com
	www.mayclinic.com
	www.diverticulitisdiet.net
	www.healthscout.com
	www.diverticulosis.org
	www.johnhopkinshealthalerts.com

	www.womenshealth.about.com
	www.mothernature.com
Hemorrhoids	www.hemorrhoids-treatment-guide.com
	www.bleedinghemorrhoids.com
	www.hemorrhoids.net/hemorrhoids.php
	www.gicare.com/disease/hemorrhoids.aspx
	www.umm.edu
Gastroenteritis	www.my.clevelandclinic.org
	www.aafp.org
	www.cdc.gov
	www.digestive.niddk.nih.gov
	www.nhs.uk
	www.drreddy.com
	www.medpedia.com
	www.medindia.net
	www.totalhealth.ivillage.com
	www.drgreene.com
Hernias	www.hernia.org
	www.emedicinehealth.com
	www.herniainfo.com
	www.herniaonline.com
	www.emedicinehealth.com
	www.medicinenet.com
	www.medscape.com
	www.goremedical.com
	www.mayclinic.com

COPD	www.gobreathe.com www.asthmapreventionnow.org www.medlineplus.gov www.copd.about.com www.getcopdinfo.com www.copd.com www.copdfoundatio.org www.mayoclinic.com www.copd.emedtv.com www.copd-international.com
FLU	www.flu.gov www.medicinenet.com www.webmd.com www.cdc.com www.flufacts.com www.facesofinfluenza.com
Pneumonia	www.webmd.com www.nih.gov www.webmd.com www.medlineplus.gov www.medicinenet.com www.mayoclinic.com
Osteoporosis	www.nof.org www.medlineplus.gov www.niams.nih.gov www.mayoclinic.com

Diabetes	www.diabetes.org www.diabetes.com www.diabetessymptomsonline.com/ www.diabetes.emedtv.com/ www.davita.com/diabetes www.diabetesinformationhub.com www.nih.gov www.medicinenet.com www.mayoclinic.com www.diabetes.webmed.com www.healthcenter.com
Alzheimer's	www.alz.org www.alzfdn.org www.alzheimers.org www.nia.nih.gov www.webmd.com www.mayclinic.com